The KINESIOLOGY WorkbooK

The KINESIOLOGY Workbook

JAN F. PERRY
EdD, PT

Associate Professor and Chairman, Department of Physical Therapy, School of Allied Health Sciences, Medical College of Georgia, Augusta, Georgia

DAVID A. ROHE
MPH, PT

Associate Professor, Department of Physical Therapy, School of Allied Health Sciences, Medical College of Georgia, Augusta, Georgia

ANITA O. GARCIA
MS, PT

Harker Heights, Texas

F. A. DAVIS COMPANY • Philadelphia

Copyright © 1992 by F. A. Davis Company

All rights reserved. This book is protected by copyright. No part of it may be reproduced, stored in a retrieval system, or transmitted in any form or by any means, electronic, mechanical, photocopying, recording, or otherwise, without written permission from the publisher.

Printed in the United States of America

Last digit indicates print number: 10 9 8 7 6 5 4 3 2 1

Note: As new scientific information becomes available through basic and clinical research, recommended treatments and drug therapies undergo changes. The author(s) and publisher have done everything possible to make this book accurate, up-to-date, and in accord with accepted standards at the time of publication. The authors, editors and publisher are not responsible for errors or omissions or for consequences from application of the book, and make no warranty, expressed or implied, in regard to the contents of the book. Any practice described in this book should be applied by the reader in accordance with professional standards of care used in regard to the unique circumstances that may apply in each situation. The reader is advised always to check product information (package inserts) for changes and new information regarding dose and contraindications before administering any drug. Caution is especially urged when using new or infrequently ordered drugs.

Authorization to photocopy items for internal or personal use, or the internal or personal use of specific clients, is granted by F. A. Davis Company for users registered with the Copyright Clearance Center (CCC) Transactional Reporting Service, provided that the fee of $.10 per copy is paid directly to CCC, 27 Congress St., Salem, MA 01970. For those organizations that have been granted a photocopy license by CCC, a separate system of payment has been arranged. The fee code for users of the Transactional Reporting Service is: 8036-686292 0 + $.10.

Preface

■ ■ ■

The Kinesiology Workbook has evolved over many years of teaching an introductory physical therapy course on the basics of patient evaluation—kinesiology, goniometry, and muscle testing. We developed this book to help our students bridge the gap between the textbook presentations of these subjects and the actual physical assessment of *normal* movement—the gap between knowing and doing.

Briefly, *The Kinesiology Workbook* offers an array of exercises related to general principles of kinesiology and biomechanics, to each major joint, and to gait and posture evaluation. The exercises include both homework and classwork, and consist of both individual and group activities.

Our teaching, and therefore this book, is based on the assumption that the manipulation of data and concepts enhances learning. Some of the manipulations in The *Kinesiology Workbook* are physical, while others are mental. All the exercises are designed to encourage students to make connections between what they have read and what they will be doing in the clinical setting.

This workbook will be of value to students in physical therapy, occupational therapy, athletic training, exercise science, exercise physiology, and physical education. It can be used to supplement introductory texts in kinesiology, functional anatomy, and gross anatomy. As educators, we know that different people learn in different ways, so we encourage students and teachers to choose the exercises most useful to them, to adapt any that can be made more useful, and to skip those that do not apply to their learning situation. For example, drawing the muscles and completing outlines enhances learning for some students but not for others. Those for whom drawing the muscles is helpful can complete the charts, while the others go on to different exercises.

The key to *The Kinesiology Workbook* is that it is designed to be *used,* not merely to be read. We would appreciate hearing from you about your successes and problems in using *The Kinesiology Workbook* and about any successful adaptations of the exercises that you have used.

JFP
DAR
AOG

Acknowledgments

Active engagement of the learner is a cornerstone of the teaching style that initiated the development of this book. For that philosophical orientation we thank Drs Carl Rogers and Jerome Bruner. For the curriculum that has allowed us to practice that philosophy, we thank Bella J. May, EdD, PT.

Many people were involved with the development of the kinesiology course for which this book was originally written. We would like to take this opportunity to express our appreciation to Dennis Hart, Rita DeFazio, Cathy Koshman, Ann Charness, Donna Zorn, and Harold Smith.

For editorial assistance in the original draft of this book, we wish to thank Sandra Eskew Capps.

Karen Waldo, David Mascaro, and Milton Burroughs in the Department of Medical Illustration and Design of the Medical College of Georgia are responsible for the fine illustrations in this book. Their work speaks for itself.

We are thankful for the assistance provided by the following reviewers: Phyllis L. Beck, MEd, PT, Leonard Elbaum, PT, Alta J. Hansen, PhD, PT, Carolyn Kisner, MS, PT, Cynthia C. Norkin, EdD, PT, M. Lynn Palmer, PhD, PT, Thomas J. Schmitz, MS, PT, and D. Joyce White, MS, PT.

In addition to the contributions cited above, the students who have participated in our classes have given us invaluable feedback. Physical Therapy classes of the Medical College of Georgia from 1981–1992, we thank you.

Contents

■ ■ ■

Preface v

Introduction 1

CHAPTER 1 *General Information* 3
   Names of Movements 3
   Planes and Axes 5
   Arthrology 6
   Myology 9
   Base of Support 10
   Center of Mass/Line of Gravity 11
   Effects of Gravity 12
   Reverse Actions 13
   Goniometry Basics 14
   Manual Muscle Testing Basics 15
   Palpation Basics 16
   Force Couple 17
   Vectors—Basic Problems 18
   Glossary of Terms 22
   Answers to General Information 24

CHAPTER 2 *Spine and Pelvis* 34
   Osteology of the Spine and Pelvis 34
   Arthrology of the Spine and Pelvis 36
   Myology of the Spine and Pelvis 43
      Muscles of the Back 43
      Anterior Trunk and Abdominal Wall
      Muscles 46
      Neck Muscles 49
   Applications 50
   Answers to Spine and Pelvis 57

CHAPTER 3 *The Hip* 64
Osteology of the Hip 64
- Pelvis 64
- Femur 65

Arthrology of the Hip 65
- Sacroiliac Joint 65
- Symphysis Pubis 66
- Hip Joint (Femoroacetabular Joint) 66

Myology of the Hip 67
Applications 72
Answers to Hip 75

CHAPTER 4 *Knee* 81
Osteology of the Knee 81
Arthrology of the Knee 82
Myology of the Knee 86
Applications 88
Answers to Knee 90

CHAPTER 5 *Foot and Ankle* 95
Osteology of the Foot and Ankle 95
- The Foot 95
- The Ankle 96

Arthrology of the Foot and Ankle 96
Arches of the Foot 102
Myology of the Foot and Ankle 102
Applications 107
Answers to Foot and Ankle 108

CHAPTER 6 *Shoulder* 114
Osteology of the Shoulder 114
Arthrology of the Shoulder 116
- Sternoclavicular Joint 116
- Acromioclavicular Joint 117
- Glenohumeral Joint 118
- Scapulothoracic Joint 119

Myology of the Shoulder 119
Applications 124
Answers to Shoulder 126

Chapter 7 *Elbow and Forearm* 132
Osteology of the Elbow and Forearm 132
Arthrology of the Elbow and Forearm 133
Myology of the Elbow and Forearm 135

Applications 137
Answers to Elbow 139

CHAPTER 8 *The Wrist and Hand* 144
Osteology and Arthrology of the Wrist and Hand 144
Neurology of the Wrist and Hand 147
Myology of the Wrist and Hand 148
Applications 153
Answers to Wrist and Hand 155

CHAPTER 9 *Temporomandibular Joint* 162
Osteology of the Temporomandibular Joint 162
Arthrology of the Temporomandibular Joint 163
Myology of the Temporomandibular Joint 165
Applications 169
Answers to Temporomandibular Joint 170

CHAPTER 10 *Posture* 173
Applications 173
Answers to Posture 180

CHAPTER 11 *Gait* 184
Phases of Gait 184
Distance and Time Variables 185
Determinants of Gait 187
Myology of Gait 188
Momentum 190
Applications 190
Answers to Gait 193

Introduction

The functioning of the human body is an intriguing and challenging field of study. The concepts and information in the field of kinesiology and applied anatomy are highly physical and manipulative, but textbooks tend to be theoretical and cognitive. This workbook provides an opportunity to use the information in your texts in a physical and manipulative manner. You will be applying information that you have gained from other sources, often bringing information from several sources together. The act of bringing together information from many sources to apply to a problem is directly applicable to the way you will be functioning once you graduate. Practical problems require practical active solutions rather than recitation.

The major purpose of this book is to provide you with the opportunity to apply information. We have purposely avoided *presenting* information in this book. Many sources already exist to provide sound kinesiological and applied anatomy information. We assume that you will use those sources to gather the information needed to solve the problems and aid in the activities presented here.

Another purpose of this workbook is to provide activities that will help you begin to develop your skills in exercise design. Many of the activities will have you determine how to create an exercise or motion or to obtain a position to accomplish a specific purpose. This is similar to designing a specific exercise to accomplish a patient or client goal.

Several activities in this workbook are designed to reinforce goniometry and muscle-testing *principles*. We expect that you will obtain those principles from appropriate texts. We have not attempted to provide a goniometry or muscle-testing text.

Chapter 1 allows you to apply general principles of biomechanics and kinesiology. The information addressed in Chapter 1 is presented by concept. Chapters 2 through 9 are related to body segments or major joints of the body. Chapter 2 addresses the complex functioning of the spine and pelvis. Chapters 3, 4, and 5 progress through the lower extremity. The hip is the topic of Chapter 3. The knee complex is addressed in Chapter 4, and the foot and ankle are dealt with in Chapter 5. Chapters 6 through 8 relate to the upper extremity. Chapter 6 details the functioning of the shoulder complex. The elbow is presented in Chapter 7, and the wrist and hand are the topic of Chapter 8. Chapter 9 presents the temporomandibular joint complex. Chapters 10 and 11 deal with posture and gait, respectively. Generally, each chapter starts with less difficult information and builds to more complex information.

In this day of women's and men's liberation, the use of pronouns can become a major issue. We believe that "he/she" is awkward, that the sole use of the masculine pronoun is inappropriate, and that text should be readable. Therefore, we have adopted a convention to deal with the gender of pronouns—the even-numbered chapters have the feminine pronoun and the odd-numbered chapters have the masculine pronoun.

The greatest benefit from this book will be derived if you go through the described activities in a manner open to discovery. Sometimes the activities represent paper-and-pencil questions; other times they are quite physical and will require some equipment or props. We have marked with asterisks (*) those items that we consider more physical activities. These will often require a partner, and sometimes a small group of fellow students.

Trust that the activity will lead you to the appropriate information. Do not spend too much time beforehand trying to "figure out" the answer. Do the activity, then explain what happened. Discussion following completion of the activity also aids in retention of the principles involved.

Many of the activities in this workbook provide time to explore with your classmates. In many instances you are asked to "design a method of measuring" something, "determine landmarks" to assess a motion, or "determine how to stretch" something. In some instances there are standard ways of doing what is requested. In some activities, we have chosen not to provide those standards, but to let you choose whatever standards make sense to you and can be defended to your classmates and the faculty. We believe that there is great value in determining a defensible method (to measure or assess or stretch), based on your understanding of the anatomy and biomechanics involved in the situation. This does not negate the critical importance of standardized methods of measurement. Rather, it emphasizes the importance of understanding why the standards were chosen. That understanding will assist you in adapting standards when a patient's or client's needs demand something nonstandard. Because of our belief in the discovery method of learning, some of the items in the workbook appear to be incomplete or lacking some information. This is done purposely to provide you with the opportunity to use your texts to solve problems as you would in the "real world."

As stated earlier, this workbook is not intended to stand without other texts; it requires other texts for information to use in completing the activities. This text is also best utilized with someone who has a strong clinical and kinesiological background. Some of the activities are best demonstrated by someone with such a background. Some of the discussions associated with items in the workbook need input from faculty or others with a kinesiological background. Do not hesitate to request clarification if it seems useful. Do not forget that your classmates are a rich source of information. In our physical therapy program, it is not uncommon to have certified athletic trainers, exercise physiologists, or other individuals with significant clinical experience to share with the class. Often the understanding of these classmates can do more to help others in the class learn a concept than additional explanation from the faculty. Talk to and learn from each other.

We firmly believe that learning should be fun. So, have fun as you jump into the study of how our bodies work!

CHAPTER 1

General Information

This chapter asks you to deal with various basic biomechanical and kinesiological concepts by answering problems and performing laboratory activities illustrating the principles behind the concepts. The chapter is organized to begin with the simpler concepts and to progress to more complex or combined ones. The later activities and problems ask you to combine information from earlier portions of the chapter. You will need outside resources to answer the problems or perform the activities. Always use your own words to explain the answers or the results of the activities. The problems and activities are grouped by kinesiological and biomechanical concepts.

At the end of the chapter is a place for you to develop a vocabulary of terms that are pertinent to the study of kinesiology. We suggest that you skim through the glossary now so that you will be aware of the words contained in it. You can then complete the glossary as you progress through the chapter, before you begin, or in any order that seems pertinent to you.

NAMES OF MOVEMENTS

1. What do you call the *movement* when you are standing erect in the anatomical position and you:
   a. *Bend* your elbow from a fully straight to a 90° bent position _____
   b. Maintain the 90° elbow bent position, but *turn* your palm up _____
   c. Maintain the 90° elbow bent position, but *turn* your palm down _____
   d. Maintain the 90° elbow bent position, keep your elbow touching your side, and *turn* your arm out so your fingers are pointing directly away from your side _____
   e. Maintain the 90° elbow bent position, keep your elbow touching your side, and *turn* your arm back so your fingers are pointing directly forward _____
   f. *Straighten* your elbow _____
   g. *Move* your arm away from your side so it sticks straight out to the side away from your shoulder _____
   h. *Move* your arm back down to your side _____

   The above movements are examples applied to your shoulder, elbow, and forearm. Similar illustrations can be applied to your wrist, hand (digits), hip, knee, toes, and trunk. The movements in the foot and ankle are typically named differently, as are some of the wrist and spinal movements.

2. Give the synonym(s) that you find used for the foot, ankle, spine, and wrist movements in the following list. Consult different texts such as your anatomy, kinesiology, goniometry, and muscle testing texts for the synonyms.

Foot
Supination _____
Pronation _____
Ankle
Dorsiflexion _____
Plantarflexion _____
Spine
Flexion _____
Extension _____
Lateral flexion _____
Wrist
Radial deviation _____
Ulnar deviation _____

3. Name the *joint position* when your limb is placed as follows:
   a. Elbow bent to 90° _____
   b. Elbow straight _____
   c. Palm turned up as in (1b) above _____
   d. Palm turned down as in (1c) above _____

4. What is the name of the *movement* when:
   a. You straighten your elbow from the 90° bent position to the 45° bent position.
   b. You bring your arm down from a position of straight out to the side at shoulder height to a position 45° out to the side.
   c. From a position of reaching as far as you can behind you, you bring your arm forward until your hand is just slightly behind your hip (keep your elbow straight during the movement).

   The point that is being made here is that your language must be clear as to whether you are describing a movement (action) or a position. The same root words can be used for positions as well as for actions, and actions must be clearly described in order to avoid miscommunication.

5. A method of specifying joint motions is the Rule of Three (McKeough, DM, unpublished monograph). In using the Rule of Three one names the movement, the bone or part that is moving, and the joint at which motion is occurring. This is in contrast to the more common method of naming motions by just movement and joint. Using this rule, item 1a would be called flexion of the forearm at the elbow rather than flexion of the elbow; 1d would be called lateral rotation of the humerus at the shoulder rather than lateral rotation of the shoulder. The usefulness of this rule will be more apparent when discussing reverse actions.

   Below, develop a full list of voluntary movements available at the shoulder and the knee, but using the clearer terminology found in the Rule of Three.

GENERAL INFORMATION ■ 5

*6. In order to move ourselves or objects through space, the angular motion that occurs around our joints must become linear motion. Observe a subject and describe the angular motion that occurs in each of the following bones to accomplish the described actions:

   a. Humerus at the shoulder and forearm at the elbow to push a book away from the body across the surface of a table

   b. Femur at the hip and tibia at the knee to pull a book across the floor from in front to slightly behind the subject

PLANES AND AXES

7. What is the other name for the coronal plane? _____

8. What is the other name for the horizontal plane? _____

*9. Use a stiff piece of paper such as the back of a tablet and place it parallel to each of the cardinal planes of the body. You can place it with respect to the planes of your body or a partner's body. This activity is to provide you with a physical representation of the imaginary two-dimensional cardinal planes. For a pictorial representation of these planes see the diagrams related to item 14 of the trunk chapter (Chapter 2).

*10. A way to visualize an axis is to use a pencil or other straight object. Place the pencil pointing at the shoulder of a partner so that, if it went through the shoulder joint, you could visualize the humerus turning on it, that is, the pencil is a pivot point for the head of the humerus. Now, with the shoulder starting in the anatomical position for each movement below, place the pencil so the humerus turns on it to produce:

   a. Flexion and extension
   b. Adduction and abduction
   c. Medial and lateral rotation

11. Name the plane and axis for each motion in 10, above. For our purposes, an axis will be named by the direction of its orientation, that is, medial-lateral, anterior-posterior, vertical.

   plane   **axis**
   a. _____ and _____
   b. _____ and _____
   c. _____ and _____

12. Give the planes in which the following motions take place:

   a. Stepping up a step _____
   b. Abduction of the femur at the hip _____
   c. Turning a screwdriver with forearm:
      As in 1c above _____
      With forearm at side _____
   d. Shaking head "no" _____
   e. Straight sit-up _____
   f. Side bending of trunk _____

ARTHROLOGY

13. In your own words, describe the three major types of joints:
    a. Fibrous joint:

    b. Cartilaginous joint:

    c. Synovial joint:

14. Of the synovial joints, which type(s) has (have):
    a. Three degrees of freedom

    b. Two degrees of freedom

    c. One degree of freedom

*15. Using heavy paper or cardboard, cut out representations, in profile, of the bone ends and part of the long bone shaft of an interphalangeal joint. Align the cut out model in the same orientation as the proximal interphalangeal joint of your index finger. Now:
    a. Actively flex and extend the middle phalanx of your index finger on the proximal phalanx (the middle phalanx moves, the proximal one does not).
    b. Reproduce the movement with the cardboard cutout.
    c. Actively flex and extend the proximal phalanx of your index finger on the middle phalanx (the proximal phalanx moves while you hold the middle one still).
    d. Reproduce the movement with the cardboard cutout.

16. Below are drawings of a joint (Figs. 1–1 and 1–2). On Figure 1–1, place arrows that will indicate the direction of movement of the convex joint surface and its shaft as the joint flexes on the stationary concave surface (one arrow for the joint surface and one arrow for the shaft). Label those arrows flexion. Next, on the same drawing, draw a second set of arrows for the convex surface and its shaft as it extends and label them extension.
    Place arrows on Figure 1–2 indicating flexion and extension of the concave surface as it moves on a stationary convex surface. Place a second set of arrows for flexion and extension of the shaft.
    Your arrows above and item 15 demonstrate a principle of movement of convex-concave joint surfaces in relation to the bones to which they are attached.

Figures 1–1 and 1–2

a. What is the relationship between the movement of the joint surface and movement of the shaft when a convex surface moves over a concave surface?

b. What is the relationship between the movement of the joint surface and the shaft when a concave surface moves over a convex surface?

c. Now put this in your own words as a principle of motion.

*17. Place a femur at a 30° angle to the surface of a table with both condyles in contact with the surface. The femur should be oriented with the femoral head angled up, rather than down (see Fig. 1–3).

Figure 1–3

Now, keep the condyles in contact with the same spot on the table and raise the shaft to vertical.
a. Describe the movement of the femoral condyles at the point of contact with the table as the shaft is moved to vertical.

b. Try the activity again, keeping the condyles in contact with the table top but allowing them to move off the spot as the femur comes to vertical. Describe what you saw occur at this time.

*18. Select a partner and have him lie supine on a plinth. You are about to do joint accessory motions, and may need faculty input for confirmation of your technique.
a. You will be examining the left shoulder so you will be on the left side of the subject with your left hand placed firmly over the anterior aspect of the clavicle to hold the shoulder girdle down on the plinth. Place

your right hand beneath the humerus close to the axilla. Grasp the humerus firmly (do not dig your fingers in), press down with your left hand and pick up with your right hand. Attempt to move the humerus as a unit, keeping it horizontally oriented as it moves. You should see the humerus come up slightly and a slight bulge appear in the anterior shoulder just beneath the acromion.

b. You have just produced an anterior glide mobilization of the glenohumeral joint. Anterior-posterior gliding are accessory movements available in the glenohumeral joint. Inferior glide and lateral distraction are also available in this joint. How could you produce these in your subjects? Try it.

c. What accessory movements can you produce in the MCP (metacarpophalangeal) joint of the index finger of the hand?

Not all accessory movements are passively performed by one individual on another. Some are produced during normal everyday activities. For example, grasp a drink can tightly and watch your fingers closely. You will see them rotating on their long axes to accommodate the pressure. Axial rotation in the fingers is not a movement normally under voluntary control.

19. Give a definition of accessory joint movement and speculate on its kinesiological usefulness.

*20. a. While relaxed and sitting, put your knee in a position that makes it difficult to move your patella with your fingers, that is, the patella appears to be firmly fixed in that position. What is that position of the knee?

b. Now put your knee in a position in which it is easy to move your patella. What is that position?

c. What structures caused the difference in the ease of movement of the patella?

You have just demonstrated the difference in loose-packed and close-packed positions of the patellofemoral joint.

d. Passively abduct and adduct the index MCP joint in various positions of flexion and extension. Determine the open- and close-packed positions of that joint.

e. In your own words define open-packed position and close-packed position.

Open-packed:

Close-packed:

*21. Standing erect, flex your right humerus at the shoulder keeping your elbow extended so your hand is out in front of you. Now:
   a. Bend and straighten your right elbow.
   b. Grasp an immovable object and bend your right elbow (you will have to move your body in order to allow your elbow to bend).
   c. Which situation was the open kinematic chain and which was the closed chain?

   d. How many and which joints moved in a and how many in b?

22. There are no muscles that control elbow movement and have a line of pull that crosses the medial or lateral aspect of the joint. Why?

*23. a. Observe a partner and determine the number of cardinal planes in which each of the following joints can voluntarily move.
   - MCP joint of the index finger
   - PIP (proximal interphalangeal) joint of the index finger
   - Knee joint
   - Humeroulnar joint
   - Hip joint

   The joints that allow movement in one plane have one degree of freedom; in two planes, two degrees, and so on.
   b. Now observe which of the joints can perform circumduction and associate that observation with the degrees of freedom available to that joint.

MYOLOGY

*24. For this activity you will need a piece of string at least 2 ft long or a rubber band and an articulated skeleton. Place the string or rubber band across the appropriate joint so that, if it were a shortening muscle pulling one attachment toward the other, the following motions would occur:
   a. Abduction of the femur at the hip
   b. Extension of the hand at the wrist
   c. Adduction of the humerus at the shoulder
   d. Flexion with supination of the forearm at the elbow
   e. Extension of the femur at the hip with flexion of the tibia at the knee

25. The string in item 24 represents the line of pull of the muscle involved. For each muscle represented in item 24, describe the orientation and direction of the muscle's line of pull to the axis of joint motion. Orientation means anterior or posterior, medial or lateral, superior or inferior. Direction of the line of pull could be in an anterior-to-posterior direction, medial-to-lateral direction, inferior-to-superior direction, or their opposites.
   a.
   b.
   c.
   d.
   e.

26. You will need a cut rubber band or straight piece of elastic for this activity. Select a partner and place one end of the rubber band on the proximal sternum. *Slightly* stretch the band and hold the other end in place on the subject's *right* mastoid process. Ask the subject to move his or her head in the direction of the line of pull of the rubber band as you allow it to contract. You should see the combined movement of turning the head toward the left and tipping toward the right and forward as the rubber band shortens.

    NOTE: Be sure to move the head to a point that brings the rubber band to its shortest length. That point best demonstrates the combined action of unilateral sternocleidomastoid action.

    You have just demonstrated the action of a unilateral pull of the sternocleidomastoid muscle. Now describe the relationship and direction of the line of pull of the muscle to the axis of motion for each of the component motions described.

    a. Rotation of the head on the neck

    b. Lateral bending of the head and neck

    c. Flexion of the upper cervical spine on the lower cervical spine

*27. From a position of sitting on the floor with your legs straight in front of you, perform an eccentric contraction of your iliopsoas muscles bilaterally. In what position are you now?

*28. From this new position, perform a concentric contraction of your neck flexors and maintain this new position for a slow count of 20. Describe the position you were holding. What type of contraction were your neck muscles performing while you were counting to 20?

*29. a. Name the prime mover for extension of the femur at the hip. _____
    b. Is it the agonist or antagonist for that movement? _____
    c. Is it the agonist or antagonist for flexion of the femur at the hip? _____
    d. Name a synergist for extending the femur at the hip. _____
    e. Slowly move from a standing position to sitting in a chair and feel the contraction in the prime mover for hip extension. What function did the contraction in the prime mover play during the move from standing to sitting?

    f. From a standing position, slowly step up onto a surface at least 12 in high and feel the contraction in the prime mover for hip extension. What function did the contraction in the prime mover play during stepping up?

    g. What type of muscle contraction (eccentric, concentric, isometric) was performed in e and f?

30. Since the prime mover for extension of the femur at the hip also can produce lateral rotation of the femur, some other muscle(s) must be active when you perform extension of the femur at the hip without simulta-

neous lateral rotation. A muscle performing this function is called a neutralizing synergist or neutralizer. What muscles(s) about the hip could serve this function for the prime mover thus allowing pure extension?

BASE OF SUPPORT

*31. Take the ink barrel out of the pen you are using (assuming you are using a ballpoint pen) and stand the empty holder on the tapered end. It should stand alone.

Repeat the procedure with the ink barrel back in the pen, standing it on the point. Explain the difference in result using the principles of line of gravity and base of support.

CENTER OF MASS/LINE OF GRAVITY

*32. Find the point where the composite center of mass is located in your pen or pencil. How did you do it? How could you find it in a classmate?

*33. For the activities in this item, you will need a plumb line, additional string, tongue depressor, tape, stickers labeled A and B, and a subject in laboratory clothes.
   a. Ask a subject to stand, and place a stick-on marker labeled A on the lateral aspect of the body lateral to where the body's composite center of mass is considered to be located. Drop a plumb line from the marker. Where does the line fall in relation to the feet?

   b. Have the subject sit on a stool. When a subject is sitting, the center of mass has moved to a point on the anterior surface of the body just above the navel (approximately). Put a second marker B on the subject lateral to this point. Drop a plumb line from this point. Where does the line fall in relation to the feet?

c. Ask the subject to SLOWLY come to standing with no trunk or hip flexion. Record what happens to the subject. Did sticker B ever appear to be over the feet?

d. Now allow trunk and hip flexion and ask the subject to repeat the activity. Be sure the subject moves slowly in order to watch the alignment of sticker B in relation to the feet. At the point when the subject first begins to rise, stop the movement and record where the plumb line from B falls relative to the position of the feet. When the subject first begins to rise, where are the subject's head and shoulders in relation to the feet?

HINT: Attach a weighted string to the lateral side of the subject's shoulder so the string extends out to the side and the weight falls to the side of the seat. A tongue depressor taped to the top of the shoulder with the string hanging down from it usually works.

Discuss your findings in terms of:
- Shift in line of gravity of the trunk
- Relationship between the line of gravity and the base of support in coming to stand
- How this activity relates to item 31

EFFECTS OF GRAVITY

*34. For the three activities listed below, decide what force is the prime mover for the action, what muscles are active during the action, and what type of contraction (concentric, eccentric, isometric) the muscles are performing. When identifying the responsible muscles, use groupings such as flexors, extensors, abductors of the joint(s) in question rather than muscle names. Do the action or have a partner do the action and palpate the muscles to verify your observations.

While standing perform the indicated actions:

a. Slowly *lower* a 10-lb weight from the flexed elbow to the fully extended elbow position.

b. Slowly *bend* forward at the waist.

c. Stand on your right leg and pick the left foot up. Hold onto a table for balance and slowly *flex* your *right* knee from the fully extended position.

Remember that you are concentrating on the movement, not the new position assumed.

35. In item 34 above, the movements performed were extension of the forearm at the elbow, flexion of the trunk and pelvis at the hip, and flexion of the femur and the tibia at the knee. The muscle groups that are usually the prime movers for these actions are, of course, the elbow extensors, trunk and hip flexors, and knee flexors, respectively. Explain why these muscles were not needed in the actions as performed. Explain it to your landlady so she understands (assuming that your landlady is naive of kinesiology).

*36. Now do the following.
   a. Place your body or limb in a position for each of the movements in item 34 so that the movement is caused by the muscle group responsible for the action, that is, the elbow extensors cause extension of the forearm at the elbow, and so on. Make sure your positioning does not allow gravity to assist with the movement.
   b. Record the position of the limb or your body that satisfied the criteria.

   c. What type of contraction was performed by the muscle(s) in each of these cases (eccentric, concentric, isometric)?

REVERSE ACTIONS

*37. Perform the following movements:
   a. Flex your hip, but keep your femur stable.
   b. Dorsiflex your ankle, but keep your foot flat on the floor.
   c. Find a way to extend your knee, but keep your tibia stable.

   Name each of these actions according to the Rule of Three. All of these are reverse actions.

*38. Reverse actions can also be accomplished with eccentric contractions.
   a. Demonstrate the reverse action of the pelvis moving on the femur with the primary force provided by gravity and controlled by an eccentric contraction.
   b. Based on items 37 and 38, develop a definition of the concept of reverse action.

GONIOMETRY BASICS

*39. Use a blackboard or a large piece of paper and place two dots on it that determine a line. Place the stationary arm of a goniometer on the surface so that the dots fall on the centerline of the goniometer. Now, place two more dots on the surface to describe a line that is close to and will intersect with the first line. Keeping the first two dots under the midline of the stationary arm, align the movable arm of the goniometer so that the second set of dots fall on the centerline of that arm. (Depending on where you placed the second two dots, you may have to slide the goniometer up or down to get the movable arm over the second two dots.) Read the angle on the goniometer.

*40. Repeat exercise 39, but this time place all four dots on the surface before you align the goniometer. Be sure the two lines described by the four dots intersect at some point. Align the goniometer arms so that they form the angle described by the two lines. Read the angle. Take the goniometer off and close it. Have a second person repeat the measurement and compare measurements.

*41. You will need a Ping-Pong ball to complete the next task. If you are using a blackboard, you will hang the ball from a string. If you are using paper, simply place the ball over an area representing one of the dots.
   Place two dots on the blackboard or paper to describe a line. Place one dot and the Ping-Pong ball for the second dot to represent another line that will intersect with the first. *Do not* hold the ball in place. Place the goniometer over the ball and its dot being sure the goniometer is in contact with the ball as you take the measurement. Measure the angle described by the two lines. Take the goniometer off and close it. Have a second person repeat the measurement. Compare the results of activity 40 and this activity for:
   a. Ease of obtaining an accurate measurement
   b. Reproducibility of results

42. Assuming that we can study the body as a system of levers and axes, state whatever principles of goniometric measurement you understand as a result of items 39 to 41. In your deliberation, consider:
   a. The definition of a line
   b. The importance of stability of each reference landmark (point)
   c. The relative importance of the placement of the axis of the goniometer versus the placement of the arms of the goniometer during measurement.
   Principles:

MANUAL MUSCLE TESTING BASICS

*43. Select a subject who is dressed in loose fitting shorts. Place this subject so that he performs an active extension of the femur at the hip from the anatomical position or 0° starting position. The movement must be accomplished without gravity resisting or assisting the movement and with the limb supported on a plinth. (Hint, you may have to assist the subject for balance.) Do the same activity for abduction of the humerus at the shoulder, flexion of the forearm at the elbow, and flexion of the tibia at the knee. In each case have the subject complete a full range of motion. How did you decide that gravity was not resisting or assisting the motions? In what plane did each of the motions take place?

*44. Have your subject sit on the edge of the treatment table with his feet dangling. Have him flex the right forearm at the elbow to about 120°. Grasp the wrist of the flexed arm with your right hand and ask the subject to keep the elbow flexed and his left hand behind his back. (Note: This is a modification of the muscle-testing position for biceps. Consult a muscle-testing text for an illustration.) Instruct him not to lean back and not to support himself with the left hand. Now, gradually pull on the right wrist in an attempt to straighten the elbow. Pull until you obtain a reaction from the subject. What reaction did you obtain?

Now, place your left hand in front of the subject's right shoulder, your palm to his shoulder, and push against the shoulder as you pull with your right hand. Pull hard with your right hand, but do not allow the shoulder to come forward.

   a. In which exercise did the subject resist more strongly with elbow flexion?
   b. In the second part of this activity you stabilized your partner. Now state a use or uses of stabilization in the performance of manual muscle testing.

*45. Select two subjects, each with the shoulders exposed. One subject should have a large frame and well-defined shoulder girdle musculature. The other should be slightly built with relatively small shoulder girdle musculature. Seat the subjects on low stools. Stand behind the larger subject and ask him to abduct the humerus at the shoulder to 90° bilaterally. Place your hand just above the elbow and have the subject resist while you push down vigorously. How much resistance can you apply? Can you break the contraction? Now, resist the slightly built subject in the same way. Could you break that contraction?

Answer the following questions:

   a. Is either subject considered abnormal?
   b. Were you able to apply maximal resistance to each subject?
   c. Define maximal resistance.

*46. a. On the slightly built subject, with the humerus abducted 90° at the shoulder apply your downward force just above the elbow, but at an acute angle rather than perpendicular to the humerus; have most of your force directed laterally rather than downward. Compare the force you needed to apply in this exercise with the force you used in item 45. Was there a difference in the amount of force you had to apply to break the contraction? Why?

    b. With the same subject, repeat the process but place your resisting hand on the humerus just distal to the shoulder joint rather than close to the elbow. Apply your resistance perpendicular to the humerus. Compare the force you exerted to break the abduction contraction this time to the force you used in item 45 and in a, above. Relate your findings in items 45, 46a, and 46b to the principles of resistance application outlined in your muscle-testing text.

*47. Select a subject who has well-developed shoulder musculature and normal shoulder structure. Ask the subject to assume the position described in item 45. Tell the subject that you will be applying maximum pressure and ask the subject to fix the shoulders as well as he can. Place your hands at the elbows and apply downward pressure firmly and *quickly*. You will see the arms go down slightly, even though the subject is strong and was theoretically prepared for the resistance. Repeat the procedure and build your resistance slowly. The arms will not go down.

    How do these findings relate to the technique of applying resistance in a manual muscle-testing break test?

PALPATION BASICS

The following exercises are designed to allow you structured feedback about the effects of your touch-palpation on a subject, and to help you learn some of the basic principles of successful palpation. For these activities to achieve their ends, the subject *must* tell the person doing the palpation what he feels (comfort or discomfort, safe or unsafe, etc.). It is much better to obtain that information from a student colleague than from a patient in the clinic.

*48. As therapist, communicate through touch the following attitudes to your subject. Do not use words and do the activities in random order. The subject is to tell the therapist what the attitude is that is being conveyed. During the activities, the therapist should compare how relaxed the subject felt under each of the circumstances.

    The therapist tries to impart a sense of:
  a. Confidence and competence while performing passive flexion of the head on the neck (subject supine with head off end of the plinth)
  b. Tentativeness and apprehension during passive flexion of the head on the neck (subject same position)
  c. Care and concern, attending to the patient during passive knee flexion and extension
  d. Being rushed and impersonal during passive knee flexion and extension

*49. Palpate, and then analyze what you had to do in order to successfully palpate, each of the following items. Remember, the subject should continue to provide feedback to the therapist concerning the non-verbal cues delivered and the comfort of the palpation.
   a. Radial pulse
   b. Acromion
   c. Radial head
   d. Sternocleidomastoid (SCM) muscle from origin to insertion
   Analysis:

*50. Palpate a contraction in the pronator teres muscle as differentiated from the wrist and finger flexors. What did you have to do in order to confirm that you were palpating the pronator, and to differentiate the pronator from the flexors?

FORCE COUPLE

*51. Connect two 12-ft lengths of rope to diagonally opposite legs of a table. (See Fig. 1–4 below.)
   a. One person pulls rope X in the direction indicated. Pull hard enough to cause the table to move.
   b. Now, a second person *independently* (first person stops pulling) pulls rope Y in the direction indicated with enough force to move the table.
   c. Describe the movement of the table when each person pulled independently.

   d. Now, both people pull simultaneously in the directions indicated and with enough force to cause the table to move.
   e. Describe the motion resulting from the simultaneous pull.

   The simultaneous pull resulted in a force couple. In this text, examples of muscles acting as force couples on bones are discussed in the chapters related to shoulder, pelvis, and temporomandibular joint.

Figure 1–4

VECTORS—BASIC PROBLEMS

The remaining problems deal with some phase of vector problems. Additional topics addressed are:

Moment arm: Problems 52, 54, 59, 61
Lever systems: Problems 53, 55, 56, 59, 61
Torque: Problems 55, 56, 57, 59, 61
Resolution of forces: Problems 57, 58, 59, 60, 61
Muscle forces and effects: Problems 53, 58, 59, 60, 61

52. Recall the definition of a moment arm. Now, in Figure 1-5 consider that points A, B, and C are the axes of motion for the vectors F_A, F_B, and F_C. Draw a line perpendicular to each force vector that intersects with its respective axis. Remember that a vector is also a line and that a line, by definition, can be projected to infinity. If you use a dotted line to show the projection of the vector, then the magnitude of the vector is not disturbed by the projection.

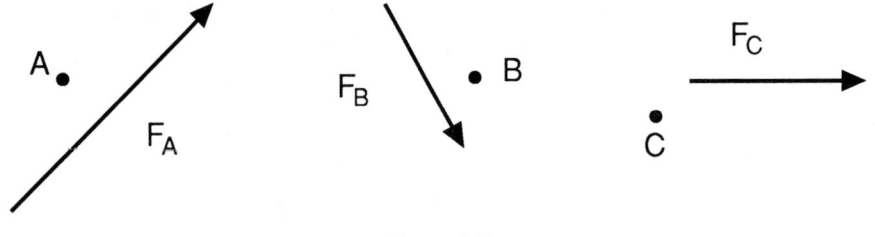

Figure 1-5

53. On Figure 1-6, label and attach three vectors to the points of application of the following forces:
    a. The force of gravity on the mass in the hand
    b. The force of gravity on the center of mass of the forearm
    c. The vertical muscle force of the flexors of the forearm at the elbow

    NOTE: Do not worry about the magnitude of the vectors at this time. Concentrate on the points of attachment and the direction of each.

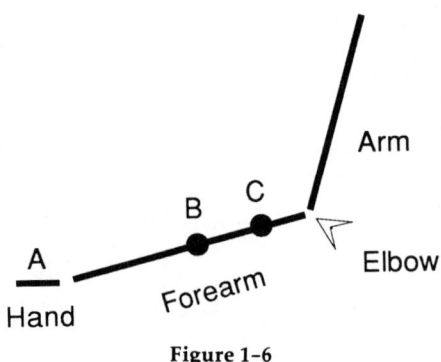

Figure 1-6

54. Measure and record, in millimeters, the length of each moment arm in Figure 1–6 of item 53. Consider the axis of rotation to be in the elbow.

    a. _____

    b. _____

    c. _____

    NOTE: For the remaining problems, 1 mm = 1 N (newton) and weight is considered to be a force in newtons.

55. On Figure 1–7, attach the vector at B that will place the lever system in equilibrium. Draw the vector to scale.

    AB = 10 mm   AC = 30 mm
    F = ?   W = 10N

    What class lever is drawn here? _____

    State the basic characteristics of vectors.

Figure 1–7

56. In Figure 1–8, how far from the axis is Wb placed for the system to be in equilibrium?

    AB = 30 mm   F = 58 N
    AC = 60 mm   Wa = 9 N
    AD = ?   Wb = 10 N

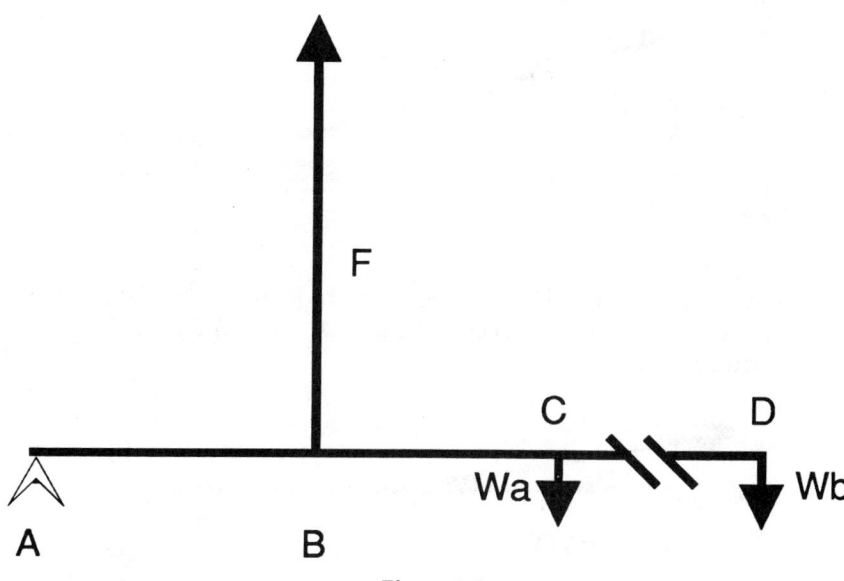

Figure 1–8

57. In Figure 1–9, a force is applied at a 45° angle to the lever. Answer the following questions.

   HINT: you will need the following table of trigonometric functions and the definition of those functions.
   Sin 45 degrees = .707; Cos 45 degrees = .707; Tan 45 degrees = 1.000.

   $$\text{Sin} = \frac{\text{opp}}{\text{hyp}} \quad \text{Cos} = \frac{\text{adj}}{\text{hyp}} \quad \text{Tan} = \frac{\text{opp}}{\text{adj}}$$

   F = 11.5 N
   θ = 45°

   a. What is the magnitude of the rotary (vertical or perpendicular in this case) component of F?
   _____

   b. What is the magnitude of the horizontal component? _____

   c. What is the main effect on the lever of the effort in the rotary component?
   _____

   d. What is the main effect on the lever of the effort in the horizontal component?
   _____

   e. What is the term given a force that produces rotation? _____

   NOTE: This drawing is *not* to scale.

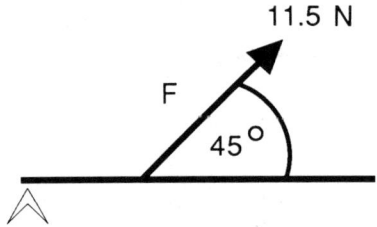

Figure 1–9

58. In Figure 1–10, force F is attempting to pull P around the end of lever AB, but P is immobile so no movement occurs. Therefore, the force is compressing P onto the end of AB by the amount of the horizontal component of F. How much is that compressive force given the following values:

   θ = 15°   Sin 15° = .259   Tan 15° = .268
   F = 100 N   Cos 15° = .965

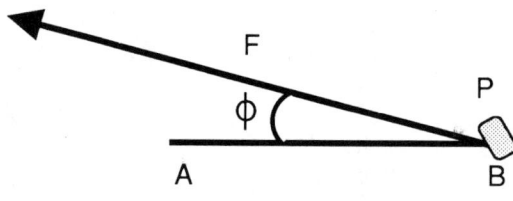

Figure 1–10

59. In Figure 1–11, the angle of pull of F is 10° and the magnitude of F is 20 N. AC = 30 mm and W = 10 N. AB = 15 mm. The lever system is not now in equilibrium. At what angle will F have to pull in order for the system to be in equilibrium?

Figure 1–11

60. Using parallelograms, compare the two force diagrams (Figs. 1–12 and 1–13) below for:
    a. Relative amount of rotary force of each
    b. Relative amount of compressive-distractive force of each
       You will not need values for the vectors to complete this exercise

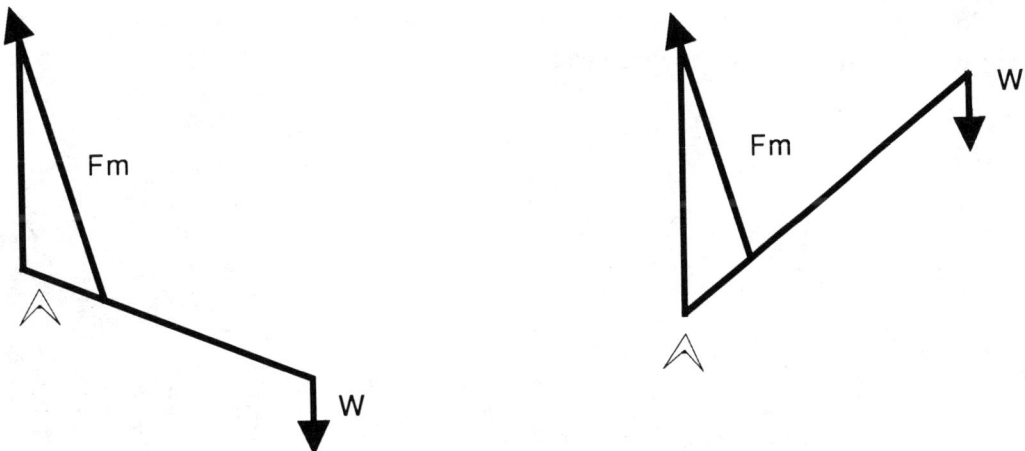

Figures 1–12 and 1–13

61. What muscle force at what angle to the lever is required to keep the system diagramed in Figure 1–14 in equilibrium?

    $\phi = 20°$ AB = 20 mm   AC = 40 mm   AD = 60 mm
    Fb = 15 N   Fc = ?   Fd = 18 N
    Angle f = ?

    NOTE: Fb and Fd are vertical or gravity forces and Fc is a vertical opposing force.

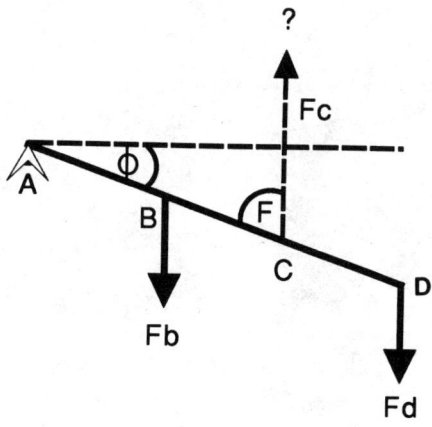

Figure 1–14

GLOSSARY OF TERMS

Below is a list of terms that we have found cause difficulty for many students. You will use some of them repeatedly in the course of this chapter, and some are terms regularly used (and misused) in professional practice. Your kinesiology textbook contains most of the definitions. We suggest you look up the definitions of all the terms now or as you encounter them in the course of dealing with problems in the workbook. Once the definitions are obtained, this glossary will be your ready reference, and will help you with the workbook.

Active insufficiency/passive insufficiency (2 terms):

Agonist:

Antagonist:

Center of gravity (center of mass):

Close-packed/open-packed positions (2 terms):

Concentric:

Contraction:

Contracture:

Eccentric:

Force:

GENERAL INFORMATION — 23

Horizontal component force:

Isokinetic:

Isometric:

Isotonic:

Length-tension relationship:

Lever:

Lever arm:

Line of gravity:

Moment arm:

Open kinematic chain/closed kinematic chain (2 terms):

Resolution of vectors:

Reverse action:

Synergist:

Torque:

Translatory component force:

Vector:

ANSWERS TO GENERAL INFORMATION

NOTE: There may be more than one legitimate answer to several of the problems. The following are the answers considered as first choice by the authors.

1. a. Flexion
   b. Supination
   c. Pronation
   d. Lateral rotation
   e. Medial rotation
   f. Extension
   g. Abduction
   h. Adduction

2. **Foot**
   Supination (inversion)
   Pronation (eversion)
   Ankle
   Plantarflexion (extension)
   Dorsiflexion (flexion)
   Spine
   Flexion (forward bending)
   Extension (backward bending)
   Lateral flexion (lateral bending)
   Wrist
   Radial deviation (abduction)
   Ulnar deviation (adduction)

3. a. Flexion
   b. Extension
   c. Supination
   d. Pronation

4. a. Extension
   b. Adduction
   c. Flexion

5. Your list should look like this: (Motion) of the (bone) at the (joint). For instance, flexion of the humerus at the shoulder, or extension of the tibia at the knee.

6. a. Flexion of the humerus at the shoulder, extension of the forearm at the elbow
   b. Extension of the femur at the hip and flexion of the tibia at the knee

7. Frontal

8. Transverse

*9. The paper is a concrete representation of the imaginary two-dimensional plane.

*10. a. The pencil should be in a side-to-side direction
    b. The pencil should be in a front-to-back direction
    c. The pencil should be in an up-and-down direction

11. a. Sagittal and medial-lateral
    b. Frontal and anterior-posterior
    c. Horizontal and vertical

12. a. Sagittal
    b. Frontal
    c. Frontal
       Transverse
    d. Transverse
    e. Sagittal
    f. Frontal

13. Since it is to be written in your own words, a preferred answer is incongruous. Major concepts that should be addressed include the following:

    Fibrous joint: minimal motion; tough, fibrous tissue joining bones
    Cartilaginous joint: limited motion; cartilaginous tissue joining bones
    Synovial joint: freely moving; joint surrounded by fibrous capsule which is lined with synovial membrane

14. a. Ball and socket (triaxial)
    b. Condyloid and saddle or sellar (biaxial)
    c. Hinge or ginglymus and pivot (uniaxial)

*15. This activity gives a concrete demonstration of the convex-concave rule. The information as to which surface is convex and which is concave will be needed prior to attempting the activity. Next, the movement of the "joint surfaces" of the paper cutouts must be observed closely to learn the direction of slide of the joint surface in relation to the direction of movement of the bone.

16. a. The movements occur in opposite directions.
    b. Movement occurs in the same direction.
    c. Your wording of the principle should have the information in a and b, above, combined with the types of joint surfaces that are involved.

Figures 1–15 and 1–16

*17. a. Demonstrates the need for slide (glide) for the femur to flex and extend on the tibia and maintain its position on the tibial plateau.
    b. Demonstrates the effect of rolling of the femoral condyles without simultaneous glide.

*18. a. Self-explanatory.
   b. For inferior glide, gently but firmly pull the humerus down along the subject's side while stabilizing the scapula. For lateral distraction, stabilize the scapula and gently but firmly pull the proximal humerus directly away from the scapula. The humeral shaft must stay parallel to the trunk for each of these motions.
   c. Anterior-posterior glide, medial-lateral glide, rotation, distraction. To see these, stabilize the metacarpal and firmly grasp the first phalanx of the index finger. Gently move the phalanx so the proximal end performs the above movements.

19. Joint accessory movement is movement not under volitional control of the limb. It allows for conformation of body parts around objects (as in the grip of the hand); deformation of the joint under stress, thus reducing the chance of injury; and greater range of motion than would be otherwise allowed. Other possibilities for answers undoubtedly exist.

*20. a. and b. As the knee becomes more flexed, it becomes more difficult to passively move the patella, especially after 30° of knee flexion.
   c. The medial and lateral lips of the patellar articulating surface, the vertical ridge on the posterior surface of the patella, the tightening patellar retinaculum, and the tightening patellar ligament all aid in stabilizing the patella.
   d. The close-packed position of the index MCP (metacarpophalangeal) joint is about 70° of flexion. This can be seen by the decreased mobility of the joint in that position.
   e. Include statements about tension in the ligaments, congruity between bony surfaces, and mobility and stability of the joint.

*21. c. The open kinematic chain is a and the closed chain is b.
   d. Only one joint moved (the elbow) in a, while in b movement at one joint affects the position of all the other joints in the chain so three joints moved (wrist, elbow, and shoulder).

22. The structure of the bones and ligaments making up the joint limit the movements to one plane, thus eliminating the necessity for muscles to control movements in the other planes.

*23. a. MCP: two planes
   PIP: one plane
   Tibiofemoral: two planes
   Humeroulnar: one plane
   Hip: three planes
   b. Joints with two or three degrees of freedom can perform circumduction.

*24. The emphasis of this activity is to note the orientation of the string to the joint and the direction of the line of the string, once the effective position has been decided. This information can then be correlated with the anatomical information available for the muscles that produce the motion. This activity reinforces the need to learn the location of the attachments of a muscle in order to determine the muscle's probable action.

25. a. Lateral to the hip, running in a superior-inferior direction
   b. Posterior (dorsal) to the wrist, running in a proximal-distal direction
   c. Medial and inferior to the shoulder, running in a medial-lateral direction
   d. Anterior to the elbow and medial to the radius, running in a superior-inferior direction, wrapping medially around the radius
   e. Posterior to the hip and also to the knee, running in a superior-inferior direction

*26. This activity is an effective means of learning about combined actions of a muscle, generally, and the unilateral action of the sternocleidomastoid muscle, specifically.
   a. Anterior to the axis for rotation running in a superior-lateral to inferior-medial direction
   b. Lateral to the axis for lateral bending running in a superior to inferior direction
   c. Anterior to the axis for cervical flexion and extension running in a superior to inferior direction

*27. Supine. Demonstrates the definition of eccentric contraction.

*28. Supine with neck flexed. Demonstrates the definitions of concentric and isometric contractions.

29. a. Gluteus maximus
    b. Agonist
    c. Antagonist
    d. Hamstring group
    e. Slowed or controlled descent
    f. Elevated the body weight against gravity
    g. (e) Lengthening or eccentric
       (f) Shortening or concentric

30. You must search for a prime medial rotator of the hip since it can act as antagonist to the lateral rotation component of the gluteus maximus action. The most likely candidate is the gluteus minimus.

*31. Demonstrates the need for the line of gravity to fall within the base of support if the upright position is to be maintained. The smaller the base of support, the more difficult it is to achieve balance since the line of gravity has such a small area in which it must fall.

*32. Find the balance point, which is the composite center of mass (where the effect of gravity is concentrated). The same could be done with the classmate, but only the point along the subject's length could be found this way. Other means are needed to find the intersecting point between the anterior and posterior surfaces of the body.

*33. a. This is an extension of item 31. The students can either experiment to find the center of mass on one another (perhaps using a teeter-totter), or simply use one of their text references to determine its location. Note that the line from the sticker falls within the length of the feet.
    b. This is a demonstration of the shift of the center of mass from the standing to the sitting position. Note that the line from the sticker falls outside the area of the feet.
    c. and d. These activities demonstrate the need for the anterior shift of body weight so that the line of gravity falls within the base of support prior to attempting to come to stand. Note that as the subject successfully moves from sitting to standing, the center of mass is shifting again, so the stickers are no longer accurate. They do, however, provide a general sense of the interaction of the center of mass and the base of support. This is a basic principle used daily in the practice of motor training or retraining.

*34. For each of the activities, gravity is the primary force causing the motion.
    a. Elbow flexors are most active, eccentrically.
    b. Trunk and hip extensors are most active, eccentrically.
    c. Knee extensors are most active, eccentrically.

35. Since gravity pulls down, it pulls the body or body part in each example in item 34 and causes the motion described. The muscles responsible for the opposite motion are active to counteract the effects of gravity.

36. Descriptions:
    a. For 34a do extension of the forearm at the elbow, but position the limb so the hand is rising against gravity, for example, supine with humerus vertical and starting with the elbow flexed. For 34b do a sit-up. For 34c lie prone and flex the tibia at the knee.
    b. The above are suggested solutions that include the positions.
    c. Concentric

*37. For now, it is important to describe the motion using the Rule of Three, because it is much more exact and aids in diminishing confusion while you are still developing the concept of reverse action. Naming the motions by the Rule of Three is as follows:
    a. Flexion of the pelvis at the hip
    b. Dorsiflexion of the tibia at the ankle
    c. Extension of the femur at the knee
       The problems lend themselves to multiple appropriate solutions, so this activity needs faculty input for confirmation of the various solutions.

*38. a. Again, the problems allow for many solutions and will require faculty feedback. One example could be standing and bending forward or backward at the waist. The pelvis is moving on the femur while gravity is providing the force producing the movement. The function of the muscles is to control the movement by slowly elongating.
  b. Reverse action is movement of a proximal (usually stationary) segment on the stationary distal (usually moving) one. Reverse actions most often occur in a situation with the distal segment fixed as in a closed kinematic chain.

*39. This activity begins the manipulation of the goniometer and the process of emphasizing the importance of identifying bony landmarks that describe the lines used to do goniometric measurement.

*40. This activity emphasizes reproducibility of findings as well as reinforcing the use of landmarks. The angle was found without the need to place the axis of the goniometer in a specific location. This is true for performing clinical goniometry as well. The reasons are based in geometry; the angle formed by lines superimposed over or parallel to the lines of an angle describe the same angle. Therefore, locating the mechanical axis of the body with the axis of the goniometer is superfluous, and needlessly time consuming.

*41. This activity works well to demonstrate that the landmarks must be stable in order to obtain accurate and reproducible results.

42. A line is defined by the connection of two points. The two points used to describe the line for goniometry are best if they are observable, stationary, and on the same bone. As soon as the reference points for the two lines are aligned under the arms of the goniometer, the angle described represents the joint angle and the axis placement becomes immaterial.
    A basic assumption that is used in this text is that the two lines that define the angle will also define the axis by the point of intersection of the two lines. Therefore, placement of the axis of the goniometer is an unnecessary step.

*43. Different solutions are possible for these problems. Each solution will have the motion occur parallel to the ground (perpendicular to the gravity line). Since the plane of motion is in relation to the body, it remains the same, that is, sagittal for hip extension and frontal for shoulder abduction. In each case the plane of movement is parallel to the ground.

*44. The most likely result is to have the subject fall or tip forward and release the contraction that was maintaining elbow flexion.
  a. The subject was able to resist more strongly with the stabilization force applied to the anterior shoulder.
  b. Stabilization allows for a better performance by the muscles tested.

*45. a. No, neither subject is likely to be abnormal.
  b. Yes, you were able to apply maximal resistance.
  c. This exercise demonstrates the principle that maximal resistance is defined by the qualities of the patient, not by the strength of the therapist. Therefore, a maximal contraction for a healthy 23 year old is different from that of a healthy 3 year old or 83 year old, as well as different between men and women (usually) and between subjects with various body types and builds. This provides a level of subjectivity to the skill of manual muscle testing that is overcome to some degree as one experiences many different subjects. One of the purposes of practicing on your classmates is to begin to define the range of "normal" strength.

*46. a. This activity demonstrates the effectiveness of the therapist's resistance applied at various angles. For reproducibility of results across time and across patients, and for maintenance of efficiency of effort, the best angle to apply resistance is 90° to the part. Force applied 90° to a lever provides a pure rotary effort, thus is most effective in attempting to turn the lever on its axis.
  b. For the best mechanical advantage and control, the therapist applies resistance at the most distal point on the bony lever. We have found it best not to cross subsequent joints to apply the resistance.

*47. In order to give the patient the best opportunity to demonstrate the available strength of a muscle, the resistance must build slowly to allow recruitment of motor units.

*48. Self-explanatory. This activity is best followed by a faculty-led discussion.

*49. For each of the items palpated, the therapist needed to know the anatomical location in relation to the surface anatomy. This can be found in a book. Then to successfully palpate each, the following had to be done:
   a. Both the subject and therapist had to hold still to be able to continually palpate the radial pulse.
   b. The therapist had to move his or her fingers around the area to determine the area or dimensions of the acromion while the subject remained still.
   c. The therapist placed fingers over the location of the radial head then rotated the radius while holding the fingers still. This allowed for confirmation that the radial head was being palpated.
   d. The therapist also had to know the action of the SCM in order to ask for its contraction. Then the contraction had to be maintained while the length of the muscle was palpated.

   The general principles of palpation operating here are: if the object of the palpation moves, the therapist must hold still to feel it as it moves; if the object is stationary, the therapist must move to feel it.

*50. In order to palpate a muscle that is anatomically close to several others, the therapist must ask for the particular action of that muscle, and then ask for a minimal contraction in order to obtain action of only that muscle. In this example, the contraction in the pronator teres will not be felt if the common flexors of the forearm are activated simultaneously. So a minimal contraction of the pronator is requested when attempting to palpate only that muscle.

*51. c. With an independent pull, the table slides in the direction of the force, as well as rotates slightly around a pivot point of one of the legs. This is a combination of translatory (linear) and rotary motion with most being translatory.
      e. With simultaneous pulling, the table rotates *only*, with the point of rotation being between the points of application of the two forces. This is the definition of the movement produced by a force couple, and a demonstration of a force couple in action.

52. In each case you needed to draw a line from the force vector to the point; the line you drew also needed to be perpendicular to the force vector. In the case of $\mathbf{F}_c$, since the vector did not pass the point (axis), an extension to the vector was needed prior to drawing in the moment arm, thus the hint that a line can be extended to infinity. To prevent confusing the magnitude of the force vector, a dotted extension can be applied in order to have the vector line pass the axis and a perpendicular line drawn from it to the axis. See Figure 1–17 below.

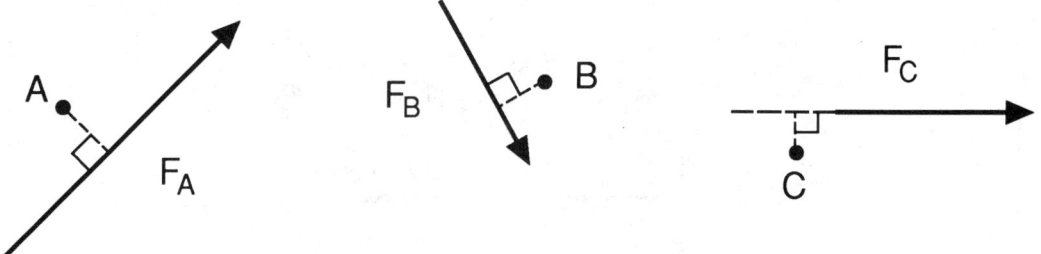

Figure 1–17

53. See Figure 1–18 below.

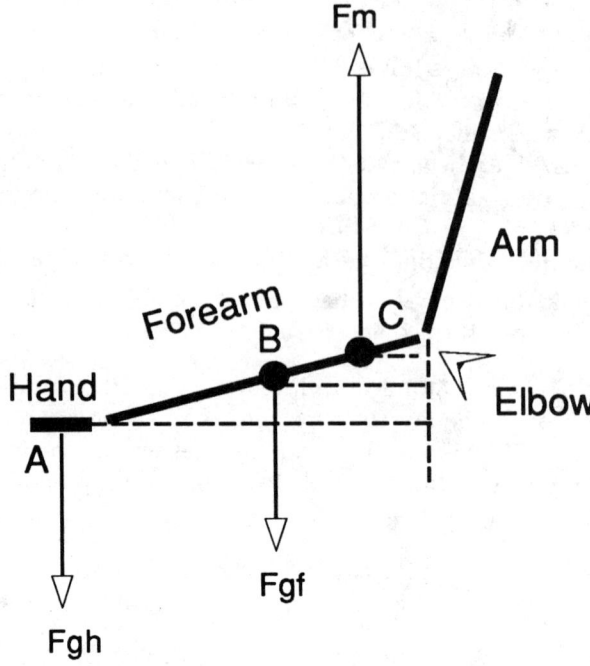

Figure 1–18

54. a. 29 mm
    b. 12 mm
    c. 4 mm

55. F = 30 N
    The lever is a third-class lever with the effort placed between the resistance and the fulcrum.

Figure 1–19

56. (AC × Wa) + (AD × Wb) = AB × F

$$AD = \frac{(AB \times F) - (AC \times Wa)}{Wb}$$

$$AD = \frac{(30 \times 58) - (60 \times 9)}{10}$$

AD = 120 mm

(See Figure 1–20 on facing page.)

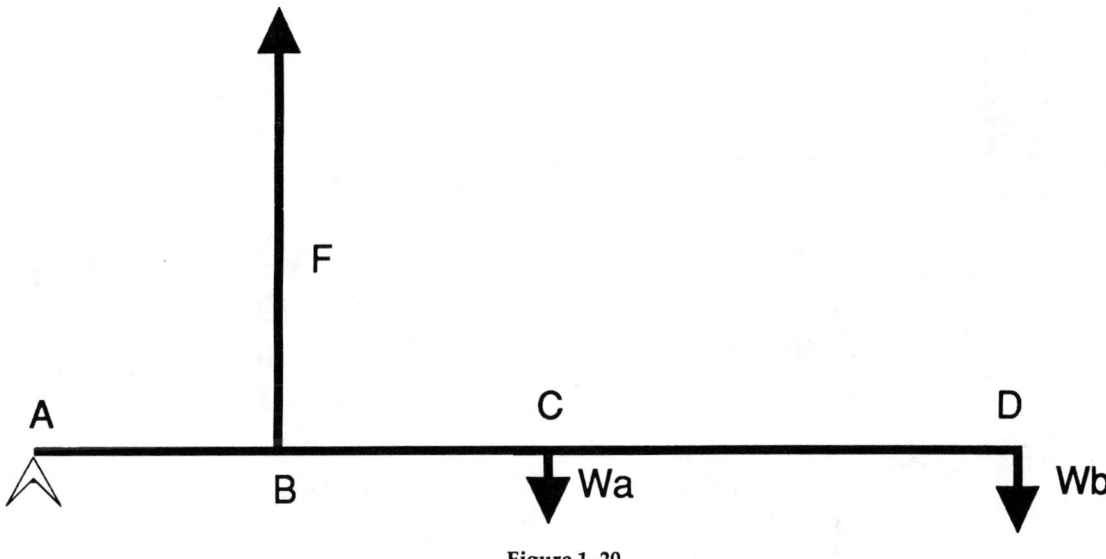

Figure 1-20

57. a. Magnitude of the rotary (vertical) component: cos 45 × F = 0.707 × 11.5 = <u>8.13 N</u>
    b. Magnitude of the translatory (horizontal) component: sin 45 × F = 0.707 × 11.5 = <u>8.13 N</u>
    c. The main effect of the rotary component is turning of the lever about the fulcrum.
    d. The main effect of the translatory (horizontal) component is pulling the lever off the fulcrum.
    e. The term given a force that produces turning about an axis is *torque* (T). T = F × d (or moment arm)

NOTE: This drawing is *not* to scale.

Figure 1-21

58. The compressive force is the component that pulls horizontally. We know that cos θ = adj/hyp = horizontal component/F. Therefore, cos 15 = X/100 or X = 100 × cos 15 = <u>96.5 N</u>.

59. The force must be at 90° to the lever so that all the force is rotary, because F = 20 and the moment arm must be at least 15 mm in order to accommodate a downward rotary force of 10 N with a 30 mm moment arm. Torque counterclockwise equals torque clockwise ($T_{ccw} = T_{cw}$)

Figure 1-22

60.

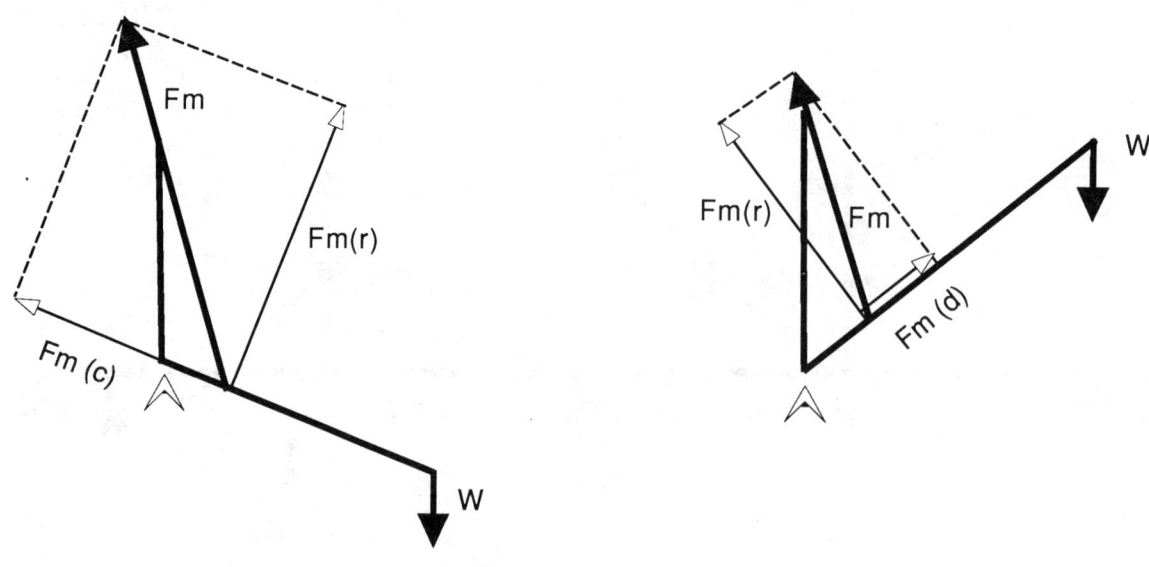

Figures 1-23 and 1-24

61. We can solve this problem at least two ways. What we need in each case are moment and forces.

Option 1

The dotted horizontal line is also the moment arm direction for the forces listed. We need to find how long each moment arm is for forces b, c, and d. We know the system is in equilibrium, so [Fb × ma(b)] + [Fd × ma(d)] = Fc × ma(c). Use Cos 20° to solve for each ma, since we have the values for AB, AC, and AD. Once we fill in the moment arms, we can solve for Fc using the torque forces in the equilibrium equation above.

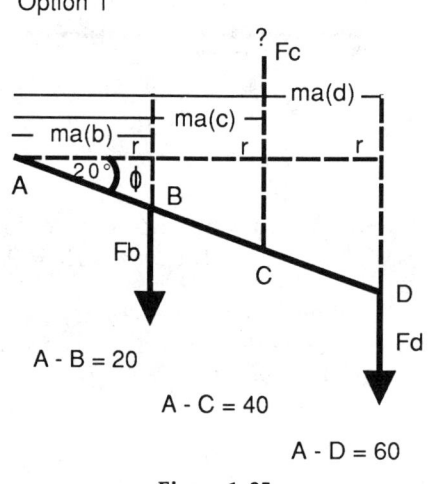

Figure 1-25

Option 2

If we find the rotary component for each force Fb and Fd by using Cos 20°, we can use the lever itself as the moment arm since it is now the perpendicular distance between the rotary component and the fulcrum. Find these rotary components and then we can solve for the rotary component of Fc (Fcr) by using the balanced torque equation. What good does that do us, you ask? Having Fcr, we can use Cos 20° to solve for Fc.

We can solve for the rotary components of forces b and d by knowing that the angle f = 70° (ϕ = 20° and we have a right triangle between the lever, the dotted horizontal and the vertical force lines, so f *must* equal 70). If angle f = 70°, then the angle between each force and its rotary component must be 20°. The Cos 20° equals adj/Fc. Now we can solve for the value of each rotary component. Having the value of each rotary component, we solve for Fcr.

Fc = 35 N
Angle f = 70°

Refer to your trigonometric tables to figure it out.

Lines Fb, Fc + Fd are parallel, therefore all intersect
with A - D at the same angle = 70°

Figure 1-26

There are bound to be other ways to solve this problem. If you have found one, congratulations.

CHAPTER 2

Spine and Pelvis

OSTEOLOGY OF THE SPINE AND PELVIS

1. Divide the 33 vertebrae into their respective categories and indicate the number of vertebrae in each segment.

2. Label the parts of a vertebra (Fig. 2–1) to include: body, pedicles, lamina, transverse processes, spinous process, and facet joints.

Figure 2–1

3. Identify the condyles of the occiput on a skeleton. Are they representative of a convex or concave surface?

*4. Describe (draw and label) the normal curves of the vertebral column from the lateral view. Indicate which are primary and which are secondary curves. Why are the curves named primary and secondary?

5. Name the bones that comprise the pelvis.

*6. The functions of the pelvis are to:
   - Connect the vertebral column to the lower limb
   - Transmit forces from the lower limb to the vertebral column
   - Support the abdomen

   On a model of a pelvis, identify the following parts or structures:

   Iliac crest
   Anterior superior iliac spine
   Posterior superior iliac spine
   Greater sciatic notch
   Lesser sciatic notch
   Ischial spine
   Ischial tuberosity
   Pubic crest

7. Define a spinal segment. Describe the exit of a spinal nerve from its respective spinal segment. Include the structure through which it exits and the relationship of the vertebral level and the spinal cord level in your answer.

8. Identify the boundaries of the intervertebral foramen. Label them on Figure 2–2 below.

Figure 2–2

9. What is the significance of a change in size of the intervertebral foramen?

10. Locate the level at which the spinal cord ends. What is the bundle of nerves below the termination of the spinal cord called?

ARTHROLOGY OF THE SPINE AND PELVIS

11. Identify the types of joints involved in the following articulations:
    Vertebral body-to-vertebral body

    Facet-to-facet

    Pubis-to-pubis

    Sacrum-to-ilium

12. Identify the intrajoint motions available to the joint articulations listed below. Intrajoint motions could be gliding, rotation, or spinning. They are not the resultant classical motions of flexion, extension, and so on.
    Vertebral body-to-vertebral body

    Facet-to-facet

    Pubis-to-pubis

    Sacrum-to-ilium

*13. The following table summarizes the planes and axes of spinal movements.

Movement	Plane	Axis
Flexion/extension	Sagittal	Medial-lateral direction (intersection of transverse and frontal planes)
Lateral flexion	Frontal	Anterior-posterior direction (intersection of sagittal and transverse planes)
Rotation	Transverse	Superior-inferior direction (intersection of sagittal and frontal planes)

Now, take a stiff piece of paper and a pencil. As you do each of the motions listed above, place the paper in the plane of the motion and the pencil along the axis of the motion. Note that the motions occur at many joints, so your placement of axes need not be specific, but rather the general orientation of the axis.

14. The planes and axes have been drawn on the diagrams below (Figs. 2–3, 2–4, and 2–5). Label both the planes and the axes.

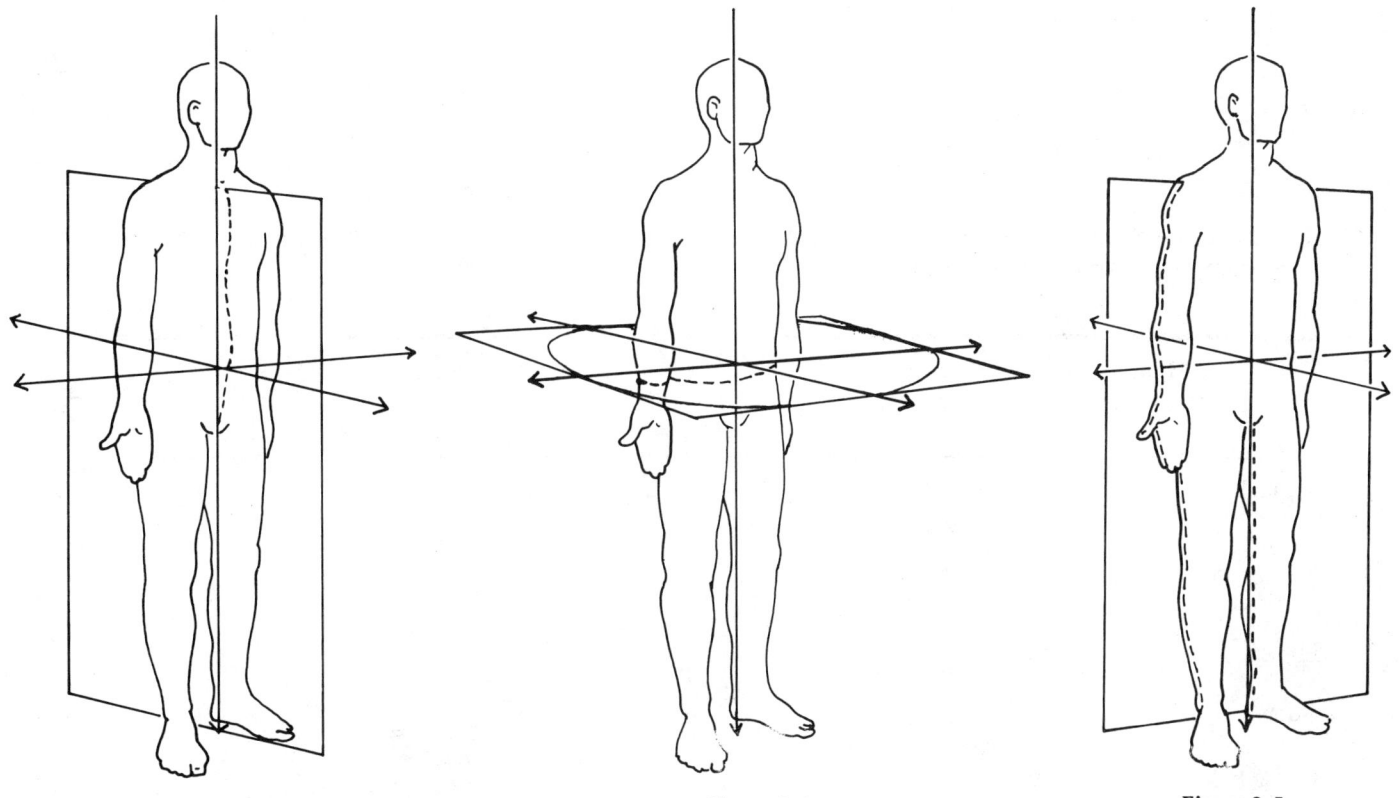

Figure 2–3   Figure 2–4   Figure 2–5

*15. Following is a summary of motions available in the spine. Do this activity in groups of five, and analyze the motions on all five subjects (more subjects will give you a broader idea of what is normal). As you observe your subjects, pick some landmarks to observe. Bony landmarks that are prominent and easily visible are most useful. For instance, the center of the chin can be useful for assessing neck motion; the acromion process can be useful in assessing trunk rotation. In your analysis and on the chart below, note in which portion of the spine most of the motion occurs. In the box representing the spinal segment where most of the motion takes place, write a 1, the next most mobile segment would be rated 2, and so forth.

Also note other observations in the chart. Is the motion smooth, is it symmetrical, is there anything that looks unusual?

What motions were easily demonstrated or observed using the landmarks you chose? What motions were difficult to observe using the landmarks you chose?

	Head (head, C-1, C-2)	Neck (C-3 to C-7)	Thoracic (T-1 to T-12)	Lumbar (L-1 to L-5)
Flexion				
Extension				
Lateral Flexion				
Rotation				

16. Complete the chart that follows for the ligaments of the vertebral column. The supraspinous ligament has been completed for you as an example.

Ligament	Location
NECK	
Apical	
Alar	
Cruciform	

Tectorial membrane

Anterior atlanto-occipital

Posterior atlanto-occipital

Ligamentum nuchae

THORACIC AND LUMBAR

Supraspinous

Interspinous — Extends from tip of a spinous process to the tip of the spinous process below

Ligamentum flavum

Posterior longitudinal

Anterior longitudinal

Intertransverse

Capsular ligaments of the facet

---

17. Identify and label the indicated ligaments of the vertebral column on Figures 2–6, 2–7, and 2–8.

Figure 2-6

Figure 2-7

Figure 2-8

18. For each of the ligaments listed, indicate which motions it will limit. Refer to Figures 2–6, 2–7, and 2–8 as you answer this question, though not all ligaments are represented in the diagrams.

   Apical

   Alar

   Cruciform

   Tectorial membrane

   Anterior atlanto-occipital

   Posterior atlanto-occipital

   Ligamentum nuchae

   Supraspinous

   Interspinous

   Ligamentum flavum

Posterior longitudinal

Anterior longitudinal

Intertransverse

Capsular ligaments of the facet joints

19. Identify the following ligaments of the pelvis on Figure 2–9:
    Iliolumbar ligament
    Sacroiliac ligament
    Sacrospinous ligament
    Sacrotuberous ligament

Figure 2–9

MYOLOGY OF THE SPINE AND PELVIS

Muscles of the Back

The muscles of the back proper are best learned as layers. Their actions can be determined by knowing specific attachments on proximal and distal vertebrae, and knowing whether the muscle is acting unilaterally or bilaterally. The actions can change significantly between unilateral and bilateral action.

Use the following sheets to aid in learning the origin, insertion, and innervation of the muscles of the spine and pelvis. For each muscle named, draw in the muscle on the sketch and fill in the indicated information on the outline.

In all the myology sections the following abbreviations will be used.

O: Origin of muscle
I: Insertion of muscle
N: Innervation (both spinal level and peripheral nerve)
R: Relationship of muscle to the axis of motion
A: Action of muscle

Deep Layer of Back Muscles

The deepest layer of back muscles consists of two groups: the intertransversarius and the interspinales.

20. Intertransversarii

    O: Transverse process
    I: Transverse process
    N:
    R: Posterior to axis for flexion and extension; lateral to axis for side bending
    A:

21. Interspinales

    O: Spinous process
    I: Spinous process
    N:
    R:
    A:

Second Layer of Back Muscles

The second layer of muscles can be grouped together and called the transversospinal muscles, because of the direction of their fibers in relation to the spinal column. Separately they are called semispinalis, multifidus, and rotatores. Again, complete the outline below (Fig. 2–10), and label the diagram.

22. Semispinalis (spans 3–5 joints)
    O: Transverse process of lower vertebra
    I: Spinous process of higher vertebra
    N:
    R: Wraps around the vertical axis; posterior to axis for flexion and extension
    A: Rotation of the body to opposite side; extension if working bilaterally

23. Multifidus (spans 2–3 joints)
    O: Transverse process of lower vertebra
    I: Spinous process of higher vertebra
    N:
    R:
    A:

24. Rotatores (spans 1–2 joints)
    O:
    I:
    N:
    R:
    A:

Figure 2–10

Third Layer of Back Muscles

The third layer of muscles of the back is the most superficial layer of muscles and can be viewed as three columns. From lateral to medial they are: cervical, thoracic, and lumbar iliocostalis; longissimus capitis, cervicis, and thoracic; and capitis, cervicis, and thoracic spinales. Note that some additional information has been requested in the outline in relation to unilateral or bilateral action of the muscles.

25. Iliocostalis
    O:
    I:
    N:
    R:
    A: Unilateral contraction:
        Bilateral contraction:

26. Longissimus
    O:
    I:
    N:
    R:
    A: Unilateral contraction:
        Bilateral contraction:

27. Spinales
    O:
    I:
    N:
    R:
    A: Unilateral contraction:
        Bilateral contraction:

Figure 2–11

Anterior Trunk and Abdominal Wall Muscles

28. Psoas major
    O:
    I:
    N:
    R:
    A:

29. Iliacus
    O:
    I:
    N:
    R:
    A:

Figure 2-12

30. External oblique

    O:
    I:
    N:
    R:
    A: Unilateral contraction:
       Bilateral contraction:

31. Internal oblique

    O:
    I:
    N:
    R:
    A: Unilateral contraction:
       Bilateral contraction:

32. Rectus abdominis

    O:
    I:
    N:
    R:
    A:

Figure 2-13

33. Quadratus lumborum
    O:
    I:
    N:
    R:
    A: Unilateral contraction:
        Bilateral contraction:

Figure 2–14

Neck Muscles

34. Longissimus capitis
    O:
    I:
    N:
    R:
    A:

35. Longissimus cervicis
    O:
    I:
    N:
    R:
    A:

36. Rectus capitis anterior
    O:
    I:
    N:
    R:
    A:

37. Sternocleidomastoid
    O:
    I:
    N:
    R:
    A:

38. Anterior scalenes
    O:
    I:
    N:
    R:
    A:

Figure 2-15

APPLICATIONS

*39. On a lab partner palpate the following items:

Posterior aspect of trunk

Superior nuchal line
Mastoid process
Transverse process of C-1
Spinous process of C-7
Spinous process of T-3
Inferior angle of scapula
Superior angle of scapula
Medial border of scapula
Lateral border of scapula
Spine of scapula
Posterior superior iliac spines
Ischial tuberosity
Spinous process of L-5
Posterior iliac crest
Sacrum
Sacral sulcus
Spinous process of S-2

Anterior aspect of trunk

Coracoid process of scapula
Acromion process of scapula
Suprasternal notch
Anterior and lateral aspect of lower ribs
Anterior superior iliac spines
Iliac crest
Iliac tubercle

*40. Objective measurement of the spine. In groups of three to five, devise a reliable system for objective, quantifiable measurement of trunk range of motion (ROM). On the chart below note the landmarks selected for measuring each segment and the technique used. For instance, to measure cervical flexion you may choose to use a tape measure (technique) and use the distance from the tip of the chin to the sternal notch (landmarks) at the end points of the range of motion. There are some standard landmarks that are used. One of the purposes of this exercise, however, is to think about and identify stable, logical, and defensible landmarks for motion assessment.

	Flexion/Extension	Lateral Flexion	Rotation
CERVICAL SPINE Landmarks:			
Technique:			
THORACIC SPINE Landmarks:			
Technique:			
LUMBAR SPINE Landmarks:			
Technique:			

*41. Now that you have a scheme for measuring spinal motion, measure each member in your group and record the measurements. What area of the spine appeared to have the greatest flexion? Extension? Side bending? Rotation? How do your measurements relate to your observations from item 15?

*42. In items 40 and 41, you have developed and implemented a method for measuring spinal motion. Could you use the same method to evaluate the normal primary and secondary spinal curves? If you cannot use the method you defined, how could you adapt your method to measure the primary and secondary spinal curves? Measure the primary and secondary spinal curves for each member in your group.

*43. Describe the effects of the following trunk movements on the normal spinal curves of a person standing:

Flexion

Extension or hyperextension

*44. Describe the effects of the following pelvic movements on the normal lumbar curve of a person standing:
Anterior pelvic tilt

Posterior pelvic tilt

*45. Compare the spinal curves of your partner in erect sitting and slouched sitting in a chair.

*46. Describe the spinal curves of your partner in the long-sitting position (sitting on a surface with her legs straight out in front of her).

*47. With your partner supine, compare the spinal curves with her legs extended and with her legs flexed at the hip and knee and her feet flat on the supporting surface.

*48. Palpation and observation of muscles. As a general rule, palpate muscles from origin (or as close as you can get to the origin) to insertion (or as close as you can get to the insertion). Refer to the principles of palpation (items 48–50 in Chap. 1).
   Palpate the following muscles, first on yourself and then on your partner:

   Sternocleidomastoid   Scaleni (anterior and middle)
   Cervical erector spinae   Rectus abdominis
   Thoracic erector spinae   External abdominal oblique
   Lumbar erector spinae   Internal abdominal oblique
   Splenius capitis   Quadratus lumborum

*49. Demonstrate trunk rotation to the right. Which internal and external obliques are working?

*50. Demonstrate lateral flexion to the right in:

a. An antigravity position. Which internal and external obliques are working? What kind of a contraction are they performing? What other muscles might also be working?

b. Standing. Do the muscles acting in this position differ from those working in a? If so, what muscles are now working? What kind of a contraction are they performing?

*51. Using Figure 2–16, draw the position of the sacroiliac joint relative to the acetabulum.

Figure 2–16

*52. Describe the effect of an anterior and a posterior rotation of the ilium on the sacrum on the position of the acetabulum. The two positions are represented in Figures 2–17 and 2–18. In each illustration, the original position is represented by a solid line and the rotated position is represented by a broken line. Figure 2–17 represents an anterior rotation of the ilium on the sacrum. Figure 2–18 represents a posterior rotation of the ilium on the sacrum.

Figures 2–17 and 2–18

Effect of anterior rotation

Effect of posterior rotation

*53. For this activity you will need two identical pieces of paper (3 in long by ½ in wide) to represent the lower limb. Use Figure 2–17 (the anteriorly rotated ilium). Apply one piece of paper with the end just touching the axis of motion in the acetabulum with the ilium in neutral (the dot). Apply the second piece of paper with the end just touching the axis of motion in the acetabulum with the ilium rotated (the x). Have both pieces of paper parallel and representing a femur in the anatomical position (vertically aligned on the page). Note that your paper represents the right lower limb.
   a. Describe the apparent difference in lower limb length between the two positions.
   b. Assume that the left limb has a nonrotated ilium. Describe the effect you just produced in terms of right lower limb length compared to left lower limb length.

*54. Repeat the procedure, but have the papers represent a lower limb with a flexed hip (horizontally aligned on the page).
   a. Describe the apparent difference in lower limb length between the two positions.
   b. Assume that the left lower limb has a non-rotated ilium. Describe the effect you just produced in terms of right lower limb length compared to the left.

*55. Repeat the procedure in item 53 on Figure 2–18 (the diagram representing a posteriorly rotated ilium).
   a. Describe the apparent difference in lower limb length between the two positions.
   b. Assume that the left lower limb has a non-rotated ilium. Describe the effect you just produced in terms of right lower limb length compared to the left lower limb.

*56. Repeat the procedures in item 54 on Figure 2–18 (the diagram representing a posteriorly rotated ilium).
   a. Describe the apparent difference in lower limb length between the two positions.
   b. Assume that the left limb has a non-rotated ilium. Describe the effect you just produced in terms of right lower limb length compared to the left lower limb.

*57. With a partner, do the following actions to simulate the motion of the cervical facets during neck motion. Each person represents one vertebrae and her hands and forearms represent the facet joint surfaces. Have one person kneel and hold her arms in the following positions:
   a. Shoulder abduction to about 100°
   b. Elbow in 90° of flexion
   c. Shoulder in 30° of lateral rotation
   d. Forearm pronation

   Have a partner stand behind the "kneeler" and have her arms in a similar position but with less abduction (70°). The stander's forearms should be parallel to and above the kneeler's forearms. Remember that your arms and hands represent a single bone. Therefore, as you move, do not change their orientation to your body.

   How do the standing person's arms and hands (facet joint surface) move on the kneeling person's arms and hands when the stander bends forward? Make sure the kneeler does not move her arms. What spinal motion does this represent? Do the right and left joint surfaces move in the same direction?

*58. How do the standing person's arms and hands (facet joint surface) move on the kneeling person's arms and hands when the stander bends to the right? Make sure the kneeler does not move her arms. What spinal motion does this represent? Do the right and left joint surfaces move in the same direction in relation to each other?

*59. Describe what happens during vertebral rotation. Do the right and left joint surfaces move in the same direction?

*60. Describe what happens during extension. Do the right and left joint surfaces move in the same direction?

NOTE: The relationship of facet motion to segmental motion changes in the various segments of the spine. The observations you have made here are for the cervical area and are not generalizable to the rest of the spine.

*61. By changing the alignment of your hands and forearms to match the plane of the facets as their orientation changes in each area of the spine, you can get a sense of what motions the facets allow or hinder in the various areas.

a. Have the two partners change the orientation of their facet surfaces to be vertical with forearms pronated. This represents the thoracic spine. What motions are limited and what motions are allowed?

b. Have the two partners change the orientation of their facet surfaces to be vertical with forearms in neutral and the standing subject's arms outside the kneeling subject's arm. This represents the lumbar spine. What motions are limited and what motions are allowed?

*62. For this activity you will need to palpate at least four subjects; therefore, work in groups of five. During this activity, you will be palpating the relationship of lumbar motion to pelvic motion during forward bending from the standing position. Have your subject standing. With one hand palpate her lumbar spinous processes. Place the palm of the other hand flat over the sacrum. When your hands are in place, ask the subject to bend forward to touch her toes, and then to return to standing. Repeat this observation on at least four classmates. Remember, you are comparing the amount and sequence of the motion in the lumbar spine and the pelvis. What did you find? At what point in the motion did you begin to feel the pelvis move (early, early middle, middle, late middle, late in the total range of flexion)? This will be the point at which you see your hand, which is on the sacrum, change its plane. Can you make any generalizations?

ANSWERS TO SPINE AND PELVIS

1. Cervical: 7
   Thoracic: 12
   Lumbar: 5
   Sacral: 5
   Cocyx: 4

2. Check your text to confirm your information.

3. Convex

4. Cervical: lordotic curve; concave posteriorly; secondary
   Thoracic: kyphotic curve; concave anteriorly; primary
   Lumbar: lordotic curve; concave posteriorly; secondary
   Sacral: kyphotic curve; concave anteriorly; primary

5. Ilium, ischium, pubis

*6. Check your text to confirm your information.

7. Two adjacent vertebrae and the intervening disc for a spinal segment. The spinal nerves exit from the spinal canal through the intervertebral foramen. Note that the spinal cord level and the vertebral level are not the same.

8. Anterior border: vertebral body and disc
   Posterior border: facet joints
   Superior border: pedicle
   Inferior border: pedicle

9. The spinal nerves pass through the intervertebral foramen, so changes in the foramen can have an effect on the spinal nerves.

10. Between L-1 and L-2. Cauda equina.

11. Vertebral body to vertebral body: amphiarthrodial or fibrocartilaginous
    Facet to facet: diarthrodial or synovial
    Pubis to pubis: symphysis or fibrocartilaginous
    Sacrum to ilium: part synovial, part fibrous

12. Vertebral body to vertebral body: tilting and rotation
    Facet to facet: gliding
    Pubis to pubis: slight flexibility of fibrous juncture, but minimal motion allowed
    Sacrum to ilium: gliding, rotation, and gapping

*13. Check your text for accuracy of your information. Have a faculty member or classmate check the accuracy of your placement of the paper and pencil for the planes and axes.

14. Check your text to confirm your information.

*15. There is no "right" answer here. Whatever you found should have been recorded. Individuals will be somewhat different.

16. | **Ligament** | **Location** |
|---|---|
| **NECK** | |
| Apical | Tip of the dens to the anterior margin of the foramen magnum |
| Alar | Two ligaments; from dens laterally to medial aspect of each condyle of occiput |
| Cruciform | A cross-shaped ligament; attached superiorly to base of occiput near apical ligament, attached inferiorly to posterior surface of body of axis, lateral attachments to tubercles on lateral mass of atlas; transverse portion of ligament is strongest |
| Tectorial membrane | Posterior surface of body of atlas to base of occiput in front of the foramen magnum |
| Anterior atlanto-occipital | Anterior arch of atlas to anterior portion of foramen magnum |
| Posterior atlanto-occipital | Posterior arch of atlas to posterior border of foramen magnum |
| Ligamentum nuchae | External occipital protuberance to spinous process of C-7 |
| **THORACIC AND LUMBAR** | |
| Supraspinous | Tip of spinous process to tip of spinous process below, from C-7 to sacrum |
| Interspinous | Length of spinous process to length of spinous process below, primarily in lumbar area |
| Ligamentum flavum | Posterior aspect of vertebral canal from lamina to lamina from C-2 to sacrum |
| Posterior longitudinal | Posterior aspect of vertebral body on anterior aspect of vertebral canal from axis to sacrum |
| Anterior longitudinal | Anterior aspect of vertebral body from axis to sacrum |
| Intertransverse | Transverse process to transverse process below, primarily in lumbar area |
| Capsular ligament | Margin of inferior facet of superior vertebra to margin of superior facet of inferior vertebra |

17. Check your text to confirm your information.

18. Apical: maintains position of dens and occiput
    Alar: limits flexion of head on neck and maintains position of dens
    Cruciform: retains dens in close contact with atlas
    Tectorial membrane: limits flexion
    Anterior atlanto-occipital: limits extension of head on neck

Posterior atlanto-occipital: limits flexion of head on neck
Ligamentum nuchae: limits flexion of head and neck
Supraspinous: limits flexion
Interspinous: limits flexion
Ligamentum flavum: limits flexion
Posterior longitudinal: limits flexion
Anterior longitudinal: limits extension
Intertransverse: limits lateral flexion
Capsular ligament of facet joints: limits gliding of facets

19. Check your text to confirm your information.

20. Intertransversarii
    O: Transverse process
    I: Transverse process
    N: Dorsal rami of spinal nerve
    R: Posterior to axis for flexion and extension; lateral to axis for side bending
    A: Side bending

21. Interspinales
    O: Spinous process
    I: Spinous process
    N: Dorsal rami of spinal nerves
    R: Posterior to axis for flexion and extension
    A: Extension

22. Semispinalis (spans 3–5 joints)
    O: Transverse process of lower vertebra
    I: Spinous process of higher vertebra
    N: Dorsal rami of spinal nerves
    R: Wraps around the vertical axis; posterior to axis for flexion and extension
    A: Rotation of the body to opposite side; extension if working bilaterally

23. Multifidus (spans 2–3 joints)
    O: Transverse process of lower vertebra
    I: Spinous process of higher vertebra
    N: Dorsal rami of spinal nerve
    R: Posterior to axis for rotation
    A: Rotation of body to opposite side; extension if working bilaterally; side bending to same side

24. Rotatores (spans 1–2 joints)
    O: Transverse process of lower vertebra
    I: Spinous process of higher vertebra
    N: Dorsal rami of spinal nerve
    R: Posterior to axis for rotation
    A: Rotation of the body to opposite side

25. Iliocostalis
    O: Thoracis: tendon of erector spinae; transverse process of lumbar vertebra
       Lumborum: sacrum; spinous process of lumbar and lower thoracic vertebrae; ilium
    I: Thoracis: transverse processes of thoracic vertebrae; ribs
       Lumborum: Lower 6–7 ribs
    N: Dorsal rami of spinal nerve
    R: Posterior to axis for flexion and extension; lateral to axis for side bending
    A: Unilateral contraction: side bending
       Bilateral contraction: extension

26. Longissimus
    - O: Transverse processes of lower vertebrae
    - I: Transverse processes of higher vertebrae and ribs
    - N: Dorsal rami of spinal nerves
    - R: Posterior to axis for flexion and extension; lateral for axis for lateral bending
    - A: Unilateral contraction: lateral bending
      Bilateral contraction: extension

27. Spinales
    - O: Spinous processes of lower vertebrae
    - I: Spinous processes of higher vertebrae
    - N: Dorsal rami of spinal nerves
    - R: Posterior to axis for flexion and extension
    - A: Extension

28. Psoas major
    - O: Transverse processes and bodies of lumbar vertebrae
    - I: Lesser trochanter of femur
    - N: Ventral rami of L-2 and L-3
    - R: Anterior to axis for flexion and extension
    - A: Flexion of femur on pelvis at hip joint

29. Iliacus
    - O: Iliac fossa
    - I: Lesser trochanter
    - N: Femoral n. (L-2, L-3)
    - R: Anterior to axis for flexion and extension
    - A: Flexion of femur on pelvis at hip joint

30. External oblique
    - O: Lower eight ribs
    - I: Iliac crest and abdominal aponeurosis
    - N: Intercostals (T-8–T-12); iliohypogastric (T-12, L-1); and ilioinguinal (L-1)
    - R: Lateral to axis for side bending; anterior to axis for rotation
    - A: Unilateral contraction: rotation to opposite side; side bending
      Bilateral contraction: flexion of trunk on pelvis

31. Internal oblique
    - O: Inguinal ligament; iliac crest
    - I: Linea alba; cartilages of lower ribs
    - N: Intercostals (T-8–T-12); iliohypogastric (T-12, L-1); and ilioinguinal (L-1)
    - R: Lateral to axis for side bending; anterior to axis for rotation
    - A: Unilateral contraction: rotation to same side; side bending
      Bilateral contraction: flexion of trunk on pelvis

32. Rectus abdominis
    - O: Crest of pubis
    - I: Cartilages of ribs 5, 6, and 7
    - N: Intercostal n. (T-7–T-12)
    - R: Anterior to axis for flexion and extension
    - A: Flexion of trunk on pelvis

33. Quadratus lumborum
    - O: Iliolumbar ligament and portion of iliac crest
    - I: Last rib and transverse processes of L-1 to L-4
    - N: Ventral rami of spinal nerves (T-12, L-1)
    - R: Lateral to axis for lateral bending
    - A: Unilateral contraction: lateral bending of trunk on pelvis or elevation of pelvis
      Bilateral contraction: extension of lumbar and lower thoracic spine

34. Longissimus capitis
    O: Transverse processes of first 4 or 5 thoracic vertebrae
    I: Mastoid process
    N: Dorsal rami of spinal nerves
    R: Posterior to axes for flexion and extension and rotation; lateral to axis for side bending
    A: Extension; side bending; and rotation of the head to the same side

35. Longissimus cervicis
    O: Transverse processes of first 4 or 5 thoracic vertebrae
    I: Transverse processes of cervical vertebrae
    N: Dorsal rami of spinal nerves
    R: Posterior to axis for flexion and extension; lateral to axis for side bending
    A: Extension and side bending

36. Rectus capitis anterior
    O: Lateral mass of atlas
    I: Base of occiput anterior to foramen magnum
    N: Ventral rami of spinal nerve
    R: Anterior to axis for flexion and extension; lateral to axis for side bending
    A: Flexion of the head on the neck

37. Sternocleidomastoid
    O: Manubrium and medial third of clavicle
    I: Mastoid process
    N: Spinal accessory nerve (cranial nerve 11)
    R: Posterior to axis for flexion and extension of head on neck; anterior to axis of flexion and extension of neck on trunk; lateral to axis for side bending; anterior to axis for rotation
    A: Unilateral contraction: extension of head on neck; flexion of neck on trunk; side bending; rotation of head to opposite side
    Bilateral contraction: extension of head on neck; flexion of neck on trunk

38. Anterior scalenes
    O: Transverse processes of C-3 to C-6
    I: Upper surface of first rib
    N: Ventral rami of spinal nerves
    R: Anterior to axis of flexion and extension of neck on trunk; lateral to axis for side bending; anterior to axis for rotation
    A: Unilateral contraction: flexion of neck on trunk; side bending; rotation of head to opposite side
    Bilateral contraction: flexion of neck on trunk; elevation of first ribs during inspiration

*39. Have a faculty member confirm your palpations.

*40. You may use any landmarks and methods that you can defend. In order to communicate with the rest of the world, though, you should adopt a standardized technique. Consult a goniometry text for standard techniques.

*41. Note that people will be different. A major factor in your measurements that use a tape measure could be the height of the subject.

   Generally the area of the spine with the greatest lateral flexion and rotation is the cervical spine. Extension and flexion are generally greatest in the lumbar spine.

*42. Any method that you choose is acceptable, as long as you can defend it. Chances are you will not be able to use the same techniques that you developed in item 40.

*43. Flexion tends to increase kyphotic curves and flatten or reverse lordotic curves.
Extension or hyperextension tends to decrease or flatten kyphotic curves and increase lordotic curves.

*44. Anterior pelvic tilt increases lumbar lordosis, posterior pelvic tilt decreases lumbar lordosis.

*45. Erect sitting: cervical lordosis, thoracic kyphosis, lumbar lordosis (mild)
Slouched sitting: increased upper cervical lordosis, decreased or reversed lower cervical lordosis, increased thoracic kyphosis, decreased or reversed lumbar lordosis

*46. Cervical: usually unaffected from normal
Thoracic: unaffected or mildly increased kyphosis
Lumbar: usually decreased lordosis due to tightness in hamstrings

*47. Supine with legs extended tends to increase lumbar lordosis, especially if the individual's hip flexors are tight. Flexing the knees puts the hip flexors on slack so the lumbar spine will not be pulled into increased lordosis.

*48. Have a faculty member check the accuracy of your palpations.

*49. The left external and right internal abdominal obliques will cause rotation to the right.

*50. a. To laterally flex to the right against gravity requires the internal and external abdominal obliques on the right side to contract.
b. To laterally flex to the right in standing requires the *left* internal and external abdominal obliques to contract eccentrically to control the motion of right side bending. Gravity is causing the motion.

*51. See Figure 2–19.

Figure 2–19

*52. Anterior rotation causes the acetabulum to move distally and posteriorly; posterior rotation causes the acetabulum to move superiorly and anteriorly.

*53. With an anteriorly rotated ilium, the lower limb with an extended hip appears longer that when the ilium is not rotated. The right lower limb would appear longer than the left.

*54. With an anteriorly rotated ilium, the lower limb with a flexed hip and extended knee appears shorter than when the ilium is not rotated. The right lower limb would appear shorter than the left.

*55. With a posteriorly rotated ilium, the lower limb with an extended hip appears shorter than when the ilium is not rotated. The right lower limb would appear shorter than the left.

*56. With a posteriorly rotated ilium, the lower limb with a flexed hip and extended knee appears longer than when the ilium is not rotated. The right lower limb would appear longer than the left.

*57. The standing person bending forward represents cervical flexion, and the superior facets glide forward over the inferior facets in this motion.

*58. Bending to the right represents right lateral flexion, and the right superior facet glides backward while the left superior facet glides forward over the inferior facets.

*59. The same facet motions that occured in lateral flexion (item 58) occur during rotation in the cervical spine.

*60. During extension both the right and left superior facets glide backward over the inferior facets.

*61. a. Flexion and extension are more limited by the facet joints than rotation and side bending. The rib cage is a major factor limiting thoracic motion and is unrelated to the alignment of the facets.
b. Side bending and rotation are more limited than flexion and extension.

*62. Flexion of the trunk from the standing position (as in touching the toes) is usually composed of flexion of the lumbar spine and an anterior tilt of the pelvis on the femur. The return to standing is the reverse of these motions. Lumbo-sacral rhythm refers to the proportion of motion that is at the hip versus the lumbar spine. In going from erect standing to a 90° angle (the trunk parallel to the floor), the lumbar spine is responsible for approximately 45° of flexion and the pelvis tilting on the femur at the hip is responsible for the other 45° of motion. You probably noted some variations from this general rule.

CHAPTER 3

Hip

OSTEOLOGY OF THE HIP

The bones to include when considering the hip joint are the pelvis and the femur.

Pelvis

1. Label the following parts of the pelvis on Figure 3–1.

    Iliac crest
    Anterior superior iliac spine
    Anterior inferior iliac spine
    Posterior superior iliac spine
    Greater sciatic notch
    Lesser sciatic notch
    Ischial spine
    Ischial tuberosity
    Pubic crest

Figure 3–1

2. During development, what three bones come together and fuse in the acetabulum to form one hemipelvis? (See Fig. 3–1.)

Femur

3. Label the following parts of the femur on Figure 3–2:
   - Head
   - Neck
   - Shaft
   - Greater trochanter
   - Lesser trochanter
   - Adductor tubercle
   - Linea aspera
   - Condyles

Figure 3–2

4. On the diagram of the femur in Figure 3–2, above, outline the angle of inclination of the femur.
   a. How many degrees of inclination does the femur in the diagram show? (Hint: Use your goniometer.)
   b. Is this normal for an adult femur?

5. In what view would you need to place a disarticulated skeletal femur in order to visualize the torsion in the shaft?

6. What parts of the femur do femoral anteversion and femoral retroversion refer to? Define anteversion and retroversion of the femur.

ARTHROLOGY OF THE HIP

The joints to consider when studying the hip region include the sacroiliac joint, the symphysis pubis, and the hip joint itself.

Sacroiliac Joint

7. What type of joint is the sacroiliac (SI) joint?

8. Describe, as best you can, the movements occurring at the sacroiliac joint.

9. Describe the attachments and give the functions of the ligaments of the sacroiliac joint.

Symphysis Pubis

10. What type of joint is the symphysis pubis?

11. Why does movement at the symphysis pubis always accompany movement of the ilium at the sacroiliac joint?

Hip Joint (Femoroacetabular Joint)

12. What type of joint is the hip joint?

13. What motions are available at the hip?

14. Draw the following ligaments of the hip joint on Figures 3-3, 3-4, and 3-5. Be sure to indicate the main direction of the fibers of each ligament.
    Iliofemoral ligament
    Pubofermoral ligament
    Ischiofemoral ligament

Figure 3-3

Figure 3-4

Figure 3-5

15. Considering the direction of the fibers of each of the ligaments drawn in item 14, what hip motion would each ligament restrain?
    a. Iliofemoral
    b. Pubofemoral
    c. Ischiofemoral

16. What is another name for the iliofemoral ligament? _____

17. Describe the open- and close-packed positions of the hip joint.

18. Which of the bursae directly associated with the anatomy of the hip is the most superficial?

*19. Palpate the following items on several different subjects:

    Anterior superior iliac spine   Greater trochanter
    Iliac crest   Posterior superior iliac spine
    Iliac tubercle   Ischial tuberosity
    Femoral triangle   Posterior spinous process of L-5
    Femoral pulse   Sacral sulcus

MYOLOGY OF THE HIP

Use the following muscle sheets to aid in learning the origins, insertions, and innervations of the hip muscles. For each muscle named, draw in the muscle on the sketch and complete the indicated information on the outline. The first two muscles have completed information as examples. The following abbreviations apply throughout the muscle sheets:

   O: Origin of muscle
   I: Insertion of muscle
   N: Innervation (both peripheral nerve and spinal levels)
   R: Relationship of muscle to axis of motion
   A: Action of muscle

20. Gluteus maximus
    O: Lateral lip of iliac crest; posterior surfaces of lower part of sacrum and side of coccyx; posterior surface of sacrotuberous ligament
    I: Iliotibial band of fascia lata over greater trochanter and the gluteal tuberosity of the femur
    N: Inferior gluteal n. (L-5, S-1, S-2)
    R: Posterior to axis for hip flexion and extension; posterior and lateral to axis for hip rotation
    A: Extension and lateral rotation of the femur at the hip

Figure 3–6

21. Gluteus medius
    O: Outer ilium and iliac crest
    I: Lateral aspect of greater trochanter of the femur
    N: Superior gluteal n. (L-4, L-5, S-1)
    R: Lateral (or superior) to axis for abduction and adduction
    A: Abduction of the femur at the hip

22. Gluteus minimus
    O: Posterior and outer surface of ilium
    I: Greater trochanter of the femur (anterior aspect)
    N:
    R: Lateral (or superior) to axis for abduction and adduction; anterior for rotation
    A: Abduction and medial rotation of the femur at the hip

Figure 3-7

23. Semitendinosus
    O: Ischial tuberosity
    I:
    N: Tibial portion of sciatic n. (L-4, L-5, S-1, S-2)
    R: Posterior to axes for both hip flexion and extension and knee flexion and extension; medial to axis for tibial rotation
    A: Extension of the femur at the hip; flexion and medial rotation of the tibia at the knee

24. Biceps femoris
    O: Long head:
       Short head:
    I: Lateral aspect of head of fibula; lateral epicondyle of tibia
    N: Tibial portion of sciatic n. (L-5, S-1, S-2)
    R: Posterior to axes for both hip flexion and extension and knee flexion and extension; lateral to axis for tibial rotation
    A:

Figure 3-6

25. Semimembranosus
    O: Ischial tuberosity
    I:
    N:
    R: Posterior to axes for hip flexion and extension and knee flexion and extension; medial to axis for tibial rotation
    A: Extension of the femur at the hip; flexion and medial rotation of the tibia at the knee

Figure 3-6

26. Adductor magnus
    O: Inferior surface of ischium; anterior surface of pubic ramus
    I:
    N: Obturator n. (and some fibers from sciatic n.) (L-2, L-3, L-4, L-5, S-1)
    R: Medial (or inferior) to axis for abduction and adduction; anterior to axis for flexion and extension (upper fibers); posterior to axis for flexion and extension (lower fibers)
    A:

27. Adductor brevis
    O:
    I:
    N:
    R: Medial and inferior to axis for abduction and adduction
    A: Adduction of the femur at the hip

28. Adductor longus
    O: Anterior pubis between crest and symphysis
    I: Linea aspera of femur
    N: Obturator n. (L-2, L-3, L-4)
    R:
    A:

Figure 3-8

29. Pectineus
    O:
    I: Pectineal line of femur
    N:
    R:
    A: Adduction of femur at the hip; flexion of femur at the hip if the femur is laterally rotated; lateral rotation of femur at the hip

30. Gracilis
    O: Arch of symphysis pubis
    I:
    N:
    R: Medial (or inferior) to axis for abduction and adduction; posterior to axis for flexion and extension of tibia at the knee; anterior and medial to axis for rotation of the tibia at the knee
    A: Adduction of the femur at the hip; flexion and medial rotation of the tibia at the knee

31. Sartorius
    O:
    I: Medial condyle of the tibia
    N:
    R: Anterior to axis for flexion and extension; anterior and wraps medially around axis for rotation
    A:

32. Obturator externus
    O:
    I:
    N:
    R: Posterior and wraps laterally around axis for rotation
    A: Lateral rotation of the femur at the hip

33. Obturator internus
    O: Obturator foramen (inner margin); superior aspect of greater sciatic foramen
    I:
    N: Nerve to obturator internus (L-5, S-1, S-2)
    R:
    A: Lateral rotation of the femur at the hip

34. Quadratus femoris
    O:
    I: Intertubercular line of femur
    N: Nerve to quadratus femoris (L-4, L-5, S-1, S-2)
    R:
    A:

Figure 3-8

Figure 3-6

35. Piriformis
    O:
    I:
    N: Nerve to piriformis (L-5, S-1, S-2)
    R:
    A: Lateral rotation (and some abduction) of the femur at the hip

36. Gemellus inferior
    O:
    I:
    N: Branch of nerve to quadratus femoris (L-4, L-5, S-1, S-2)
    R: Posterior and superior to the axis for lateral rotation
    A:

37. Gemellus superior
    O: Outer surface of ischial spine
    I:
    N:
    R:
    A: Lateral rotation (and some abduction) of the femur at the hip

38. Tensor fascia lata
    O:
    I: Iliotibial tract. (Note that this muscle does not attach directly to the bone.)
    N:
    R:
    A:

Figure 3-6

Figure 3-7

39. Iliopsoas
    O: Iliacus: superior iliac fossa; inner lip of iliac crest; base of sacrum
    Psoas major: transverse processes of all lumbar vertebrae; sides of bodies and discs of last thoracic and all lumbar vertebrae
    I:
    N:
    R:
    A:

40. Rectus femoris
    O:
    I:
    N:
    R:
    A:

Figure 3-8

APPLICATIONS

*41. Select a subject dressed in shorts. Have the subject perform the combined action of adduction of the femur at the hip with flexion and medial rotation of the tibia at the knee.
   a. Palpate the muscle primarily responsible for this combined action.
   b. How is this muscle affected by knee flexion during hip adduction?

   c. Demonstrate on a laboratory partner how you would test for tightness in this muscle.

*42. During normal gait, the gluteus medius mainly works in reverse action. Demonstrate a gait pattern associated with a weak or absent right gluteus medius.
   a. Discuss how a patient may reduce the torque produced by gravitational force on the center of mass in order to compensate for weakness of the gluteus medius.

   b. On Figure 3-9, draw the vectors showing the relationship of forces acting on the hip joint during single limb support.

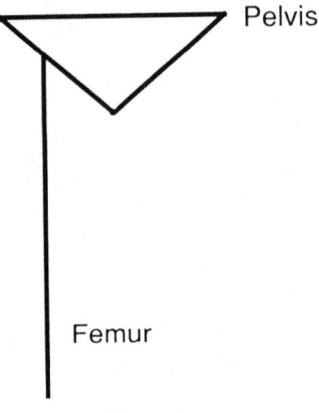

Figure 3-9

*43. In a standing position, demonstrate the effect of bilateral tight iliopsoas on hip joint position.
   a. Now demonstrate the same muscle tightness in the supine position.
   b. Describe the position of the lumbar spine when lying supine with thighs on the table and demonstrating the effect of tight iliopsoas.

   c. Develop a kinesiological rationale for what you have described in b.

*44. Which muscles form a force couple by producing forces anterior and posterior to the hip joint to cause a posterior pelvic tilt?

   a. In standing, assume a posteriorly tilted pelvis.
   b. Describe the movement of the hip joint as you performed the tilt and the position of the lumbar spine once you have assumed the position.

   c. Describe how, in a closed kinematic chain, movement of the pelvis on the hip affects the posture of the lumbar spine.

   d. What type of action is movement of the pelvis on the femur?

*45. Position your partner's lower extremity so that passive insufficiency of the hamstrings limits the range of motion of flexion of the femur at the hip.

*46. Position your partner's lower extremity so that passive insufficiency of the rectus femoris limits the range of motion of extension of the femur at the hip.

47. a. Discuss the interaction of the hip and knee joint positions to avoid active insufficiency when the hamstrings or the rectus femoris are actively contracting. In your discussion, include the effects of joint position on active insufficiency of each of the muscles.

   b. Discuss the interaction of the hip and knee joint positions to avoid passive insufficiency when the hamstrings or the rectus femoris are tight. In your discussion, include the effects of joint position on passive insufficiency of each of the muscles.

c. Describe the elegance of normal lower extremity movement that avoids active and passive insufficiency by maintaining a favorable length-tension relationship in the hamstrings and rectus femoris. Elegance is efficiency and simplicity in movement.

*48. Devise and perform a method of stretching the gluteus maximus without interference from the hamstrings.

49. Describe the motion resulting from an active contraction of the gluteus maximus without concurrent contraction of the gluteus minimus. Explain your answer.

*50. Perform a flexibility test for the hip flexors that differentiates between tightness of the iliopsoas and tightness of the rectus femoris.

51. An athlete has a bruise over the ASIS (anterior superior iliac spine). What active muscle contractions could be most painful?

*52. Position your partner to muscle test the iliopsoas so that there will be minimal contribution from the rectus femoris to the strength of the movement.

53. The lesser trochanter of the femur is avulsed from the shaft of the femur as a large jagged fragment that retains its muscle attachment(s). What reverse action could be particularly painful? Explain your answer.

*54. Mimic the standing posture of an individual with bilateral paralysis of the gluteus maximus. What is the biomechanical explanation for the posture you assumed; that is, how does this posture compensate for paralyzed gluteus maximus muscles?

*55. While standing on your left lower limb, rotate your pelvis to the left (counterclockwise) in the horizontal plane. In what position is the left hip at the end of the rotation?

*56. While standing on both lower limbs, rotate your pelvis to the right (clockwise). In what rotated position is each hip at the end of the pelvic rotation?

*57. Stand on your right lower limb on a step stool. This will allow the left limb to swing freely below the pelvis. Start with your left hip extended and the knee flexed (your foot should be well behind you). Now, swing the entire limb forward with flexion of the femur at the hip and extension of the tibia at the knee. *Actively* slow the rate of swing at the hip and the knee before the end range is reached.
   a. What muscles did you use to slow the rate of swing at the hip? At the knee?

   b. What type of contraction did the muscles perform to slow the swinging limb?

ANSWERS TO HIP

1. Check your text and have a faculty member confirm your information.

2. The three bones that fuse to comprise the pelvis are the ilium, ischium, and pubis.

3. Check your text and have a faculty member confirm your information.

4. The angle of inclination is between the neck and shaft of the femur in the frontal plane.
    a. 122° of inclination
    b. yes

5. Position the femur so you are viewing it along the long axis and so the femoral condyles are parallel to a reference line. The easiest way to accomplish these position criteria is to lay the femur on a table top with the anterior surface up and both condyles in contact with the table top.

6. Femoral anteversion and retroversion refer to the orientation of the neck of the femur to the shaft. The orientation is in the horizontal plane. Anteversion is a twisting of the shaft so that the neck and head of the femur point more anteriorly than normally in respect to the shaft. Retroversion has the head and neck pointing more posteriorly than normally.

7. The SI joint is part synovial and part fibrous.

8. A small amount of nutation or nodding of the sacrum occurs on the ilia. Anterior nodding opens the pelvic outlet and posterior nodding opens the pelvic inlet.

9. The *ventral and dorsal sacroiliac ligaments* attach the lateral sacrum to the medial ilium at the posterior iliac crest and posterior inferior and superior iliac spines.
    The *interosseous sacroiliac ligament* lies under the dorsal sacroiliac ligament connecting the lateral sacrum with the medial ilium. It is the strongest of the ligaments.
    The *sacrotuberous ligament* connects the posterior iliac spine, lateral sacrum, and coccyx to the ischial tuberosity. The *sacrospinous ligament* connects the lateral sacrum and coccyx to the spine of the ischium.
    All these ligaments serve to stabilize the weight-bearing sacroiliac joints, and thus transfer the force of the body weight to the lower extremities and the reaction forces of the ground from the lower extremities through the ilia to the sacrum and trunk.

10. The symphysis pubis is a fibrocartilaginous joint.

11. Both joints move concurrently because the pelvis is a ring, forming a closed kinematic chain. Whenever a movement of the ilium occurs at one end of the ring, movement also occurs at the other end.

12. The hip joint is a diarthrodial ball and socket joint.

13. Flexion and extension; adduction and abduction; medial and lateral rotation; circumduction.

14. Check your text and have a faculty member confirm your information.

15. a. Iliofemoral ligament restricts extension.
    b. Pubofemoral ligament restricts extension and abduction.
    c. Ischiofemoral ligament restricts extension.

16. Another name for the iliofemoral ligament is the Y ligament of Bigelow.

17. The open-packed position of the hip is flexion and lateral rotation of the femur at the hip. The close-packed position is extension and medial rotation of the femur at the hip.

18. The most superficial bursa of the hip is the trochanteric bursa between the attachment of the gluteus maximus on the iliotibial tract and the greater trochanter.

*19. The standard kinesiology, anatomy, or muscle-testing text should allow completion of this activity. Faculty confirmation of the palpations is helpful.

20. Gluteus maximus: answers given in text.

21. Gluteus medius: answers given in text.

22. Gluteus minimus
    O: Posterior and outer surface of ilium
    I: Greater trochanter of the femur (anterior aspect)
    N: Superior gluteal n. (L-4, L-5, S-1)
    R: Lateral (or superior) to axis for abduction and adduction; anterior to axis for rotation
    A: Abduction and medial rotation of the femur at the hip

23. Semitendinosus
    O: Ischial tuberosity
    I: Anteromedial surface of proximal tibia
    N: Tibial portion of sciatic n. (L-4, L-5, S-1, S-2)
    R: Posterior to axes for both hip flexion and extension and knee flexion and extension; medial to axis for tibial rotation
    A: Extension of the femur at the hip; flexion and medial rotation of the tibia at the knee

24. Biceps femoris
    O: Long head: Ischial tuberosity
       Short head: Linea aspera
    I: Lateral aspect of head of fibula; lateral epicondyle of tibia
    N: Tibial portion of sciatic n. (L-5, S-1, S-2)
    R: Posterior to axes for both hip flexion and extension and knee flexion and extension; lateral to axis for tibial rotation
    A: Extension of the femur at the hip; flexion and lateral rotation of the tibia at the knee

25. Semimembranosus
    O: Ischial tuberosity
    I: Posteromedial aspect of medial epicondyle of tibia
    N: Tibial portion of sciatic n. (L-4, L-5, S-1, S-2)
    R: Posterior to axes for both hip flexion and extension and knee flexion and extension; medial to axis for tibial rotation
    A: Extension of the femur at the hip; flexion and medial rotation of the tibia at the knee

26. Adductor magnus
    O: Inferior surface of ischium; anterior surface of pubic ramus
    I: Linea aspera; adductor tubercle
    N: Obturator n. and some fibers from sciatic n. (L-2, L-3, L-4, L-5, S-1)
    R: Medial (or inferior) to axis for abduction and adduction; anterior to axis for flexion and extension (upper fibers); posterior to axis for flexion and extension (lower fibers)
    A: Adduction of the femur at the hip; flexion of the femur at the hip if femur is laterally rotated; extension of the femur at the hip if femur is medially rotated

27. Adductor brevis
    O: Inferior ramus of pubis
    I: Femur, distal to lesser trochanter and continuing to linea aspera
    N: Obturator n. (L-2, L-3, L-4)
    R: Medial and inferior to axis for abduction and adduction
    A: Adduction of the femur at the hip

28. Adductor longus
    O: Anterior pubis between crest and symphysis
    I: Linea aspera of femur
    N: Obturator n. (L-2, L-3, L-4)
    R: Medial and inferior to axis for abduction and adduction; anterior to axis for flexion and extension
    A: Adduction of the femur at the hip; flexion of the femur at the hip

29. Pectineus
    O: Pubic tubercle
    I: Pectineal line of femur
    N: Femoral n. (L-2, L-3, L-4)
    R: Medial and inferior to axis for abduction and adduction; anterior to axis for flexion and extension
    A: Adduction of the femur at the hip; flexion of the femur at the hip if the femur is laterally rotated; lateral rotation of the femur at the hip

30. Gracilis
    O: Arch of symphysis pubis
    I: Medial surface of tibia distal to condyle
    N: Obturator n. (L-2, L-3, L-4)
    R: Medial (or inferior) to axis for abduction and adduction; posterior to axis for flexion and extension of tibia at the knee; anterior and medial to axis for rotation of the tibia at the knee
    A: Adduction of the femur at the hip; flexion and medial rotation of the tibia at the knee

31. Sartorius
    O: Anterior superior iliac spine
    I: Medial condyle of the tibia
    N: Femoral n. (L-2, L-3, L-4)
    R: Anterior to axis for flexion and extension; anterior and wraps medially around axis for rotation
    A: Flexion and lateral rotation of the femur at the hip

32. Obturator externus
    O: Medial side of obturator foramen; medial outer surface of obturator membrane; pubic and ischial rami
    I: Posterior surface of femoral neck
    N: Obturator n. (L-3, L-4)
    R: Posterior and wraps around axis for rotation
    A: Lateral rotation of the femur at the hip

33. Obturator internus
    O: Obturator foramen (inner margin); superior aspect of greater sciatic foramen
    I: Through lesser sciatic notch; proceeds to medial surface of greater trochanter
    N: Nerve to obturator internus (L-5, S-1, S-2)
    R: Posterior to the axis for rotation
    A: Lateral rotation of the femur at the hip

34. Quadratus femoris
    O: Ischial tuberosity
    I: Intertubercular line of femur
    N: Nerve to quadratus femoris (L-4, L-5, S-1, S-2)
    R: Posterior to the axis for rotation
    A: Lateral rotation of the femur at the hip

35. Piriformis
    O: Anterior sacrum and greater sciatic notch
    I: Upper portion of greater trochanter
    N: Nerve to piriformis (L-5, S-1, S-2)
    R: Posterior to the axis for rotation
    A: Lateral rotation (and some abduction) of the femur at the hip

36. Gemellus inferior
    O: Ischial tuberosity
    I: Greater trochanter
    N: Branch of nerve to quadratus femoris (L-4, L-5, S-1, S-2)
    R: Posterior and superior to the axis for rotation
    A: Lateral rotation (and some abduction) of the femur at the hip

37. Gemellus superior
    O: Outer surface of ischial spine
    I: Greater trochanter
    N: Branch of nerve to obturator internus (L-5, S-1, S-2)
    R: Posterior and wraps around axis for rotation
    A: Lateral rotation (and some abduction) of the femur at the hip

38. Tensor fascia lata
    O: Anterior superior iliac spine
    I: Iliotibial tract (note that this muscle does not attach directly to bone)
    N: Superior gluteal n. (L-4, L-5, S-1)
    R: Anterior to axis for flexion and extension; anterior and lateral to axis for rotation
    A: Flexion of femur at the hip; medial rotation of femur at the hip

39. Iliopsoas
    O: Iliacus: superior iliac fossa, inner lip of iliac crest; base of sacrum
       Psoas major: transverse processes of all lumbar vertebrae; sides of bodies and discs of last thoracic and all lumbar vertebrae
    I: Iliacus: tendon of the psoas major; distal to the lesser trochanter
       Psoas major: lesser trochanter
    N: Iliacus: branches from the femoral n. (L-1, L-2, L-3, L-4)
       Psoas major: branches directly from the lumbar plexus (L-1, L-2, L-3, L-4)
    R: Anterior to the axis for flexion and extension
    A: Flexion of the femur at the hip

40. Rectus femoris
    O: Anterior inferior iliac spine
    I: Base of the patella and from there to the tibial tuberosity
    N: Femoral n. (L-2, L-3, L-4)
    R: Anterior to the axes for flexion and extension of the femur at the hip and flexion and extension of the tibia at the knee
    A: Flexion of the femur at the hip and extension of the tibia at the knee

*41. The gracilis adducts the hip and produces slight flexion and medial rotation of the tibia at the knee.
    a. Consult your texts for palpation locations and confirm with a faculty member.
    b. The muscle is weakened by knee flexion during adduction of the femur at the hip. Since it shortens with both movements, it becomes actively insufficient when both movements occur simultaneously.
    c. The learner should find a method to simultaneously abduct the hip and extend the knee. This position will produce passive insufficiency in the muscle. This exercise can assist the learner in acquiring the skill of differentiating between tightness in one-joint and two-joint muscles, for example, tightness in the one-joint adductors (abduction with knees flexed) and the two-joint adductor (as above).

*42. With weakness or paralysis of the right gluteus medius there is an exaggerated drop of the pelvis on the left side during stance on the right.
    a. Once the learners have tried this activity, a visual representation of this gait pattern will likely be necessary to provide the learners a reference from which to reproduce the gait pattern. This can be provided by the faculty, a fellow student with clinical experience, or video tape. Demonstrate how the patient may produce a lateral lurch of the trunk over the stance limb.

b.

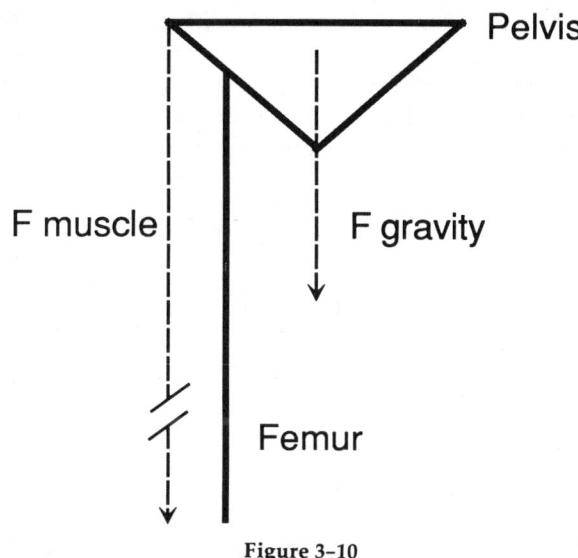

Figure 3–10

*43. The learner assumes a position of increased lumbar lordosis, assuming the thoracic spine remains vertical. The exercise is meant to reinforce the effect of a tight iliopsoas muscle on trunk posture.

    a and b. Now, in the supine position, the femurs may come off the table to hide the effect on the lumbar spine. If not, then the increased lordosis can be seen easily with increased space between the lumbar spine and the table.

    c. Since the proximal attachment for the iliopsoas is on the ilium and lumbar spine, if the muscle shortens with the femur remaining stationary the pelvis and lumbar spine move anteriorly (flex) at the hip. This is anterior pelvic tilt and increases the lumbar lordosis.

*44. Anteriorly, the abdominals attach to the pubic rami and posteriorly the hamstrings to the ischial tuberosity and the gluteus maximus to the sacrum. Together, they produce posterior pelvic tilt when moving the pelvis on the femur (closed kinematic chain).

    a. Again, a visual demonstration may be necessary to allow the learners to successfully reproduce the posterior pelvic tilt.

    b. The anterior angle of the hip joint opens during a posterior pelvic tilt; thus this is extension of the hip, which decreases the lumbar lordosis.

    c. In a closed kinematic chain, most easily seen with the femurs stationary, movement of the pelvis at the hip simultaneously produces movement at the lumbar spine. Anterior pelvic tilt produces increased lumbar lordosis (extension of the lumbar spine), and posterior pelvic tilt produces decreased lumbar lordosis (flexion of the lumbar spine). A visual reproduction of this action with a disarticulated skeletal spine is usually helpful in the explanation.

    d. Anterior and posterior pelvic tilt are examples of reverse actions with the proximal attachment moving and the distal attachment stationary.

*45. This is to demonstrate the interdependence of joint action on a two-joint muscle. This item can also be used to examine the effect of tight hamstrings on low back posture. The effect will be emphasized if the knee is straight during a passive straight leg raise. This activity may lead into a discussion of what postural changes to look for when examining for hamstring tightness. It can also facilitate a discussion of the larger concept of a tight or contracting muscle producing postural effects at remote joints.

*46. The same issues as addressed in item 45 are reinforced here. The hip must be extended with the knee flexed.

 47. a. During strong active contraction of the hamstrings in their function as hip extensors, the concurrent joint movements are knee extension with hip extension. With contraction of the rectus femoris in its role as a hip flexor, the concurrent joint movements are knee flexion with hip flexion. In each of these movements,

the knee joint motion compensates for the shortening of the muscle at the hip, that is, as the hamstrings shorten during hip extension, they are being lengthened at the knee by knee extension.

    b. Since the hamstrings cross the hip and the knee posteriorly, tightness in the hamstrings will limit hip flexion and knee extension. The maximum effect can be seen if these movements are produced simultaneously, as in a straight leg raise. Since the rectus femoris crosses the hip and knee anteriorly, the reciprocal relationship is represented.

    c. There is a relationship between the rectus femoris and the hamstrings in action and in joint position for active and passive insufficiency. The combined joint action that avoids *passive insufficiency* in the *hamstrings* during hip flexion (flexion of the knee with flexion of the hip) also avoids *active insufficiency* in the *rectus femoris* in its function as a hip flexor. The position producing active insufficiency for one (thus to be avoided) produces passive insufficiency for the other, so postures that avoid active insufficiency for one muscle simultaneously avoid passive insufficiency for the other.

*48. Several solutions are undoubtedly possible. One option is to lie supine, flex the knee and flex the hip. Knee flexion puts the hamstrings on slack, thus any muscle tightness felt in hip flexion with the knee flexed is most likely tightness in the gluteus maximus.

49. The result of a contraction of the gluteus maximus without contraction of the gluteus minimus would be extension with lateral rotation of the femur at the hip. The medial rotation provided by a simultaneous contraction of the gluteus minimus neutralizes the lateral rotation component of the gluteus maximus allowing pure extension.

*50. The critical item here is to stabilize the pelvis while measuring unilateral passive extension of the femur at the hip; once with the knee flexed and once with the knee extended. This activity is meant to reinforce principles of two-joint muscles, as well as demonstrate the clinical significance of the effect two-joint versus one-joint muscles have on joint motion.

51. Since the tensor fascia lata and sartorius attach to the ASIS, their actions will be most painful.

*52. To limit the participation of the rectus femoris in active flexion of the femur at the hip, put the limb in a position in which the rectus femoris is at an inefficient length for contraction (is actively insufficient), then ask for an active hip flexion contraction. The muscle left to perform the motion is mainly the iliopsoas.

53. The reverse action that is painful is coming to sit from lying because the iliopsoas pulls its attachment on the lesser trochanter. This attachment is now a jagged fragment being pulled by the muscle contraction into the pelvic cavity.

*54. The position assumed will be with both hips in extension past 0°. This places the line of gravity for the trunk behind the hip joint, thus gravity produces a posterior moment of rotation at the hip. This force produces extension of the pelvis at the hip which had been the role of the gluteus maximus. The iliofemoral ligament provides the main resistance to stop further extension, but the pubofemoral and ischiofemoral ligaments of the hip also become tight as the joint moves toward the close-packed position.

*55. The hip ends up in medial rotation, that is, the femur is medially rotated on the pelvis.

*56. The left femur is now laterally rotated at the hip and the right femur is medially rotated at the hip.

*57. a. The muscles used were the gluteus maximus at the hip and hamstrings at the hip and the knee.
    b. They performed an eccentric contraction. This information will be specifically utilized in the chapter on gait.

CHAPTER 4

Knee

OSTEOLOGY OF THE KNEE

1. On the pictures below, label the following bony landmarks and place an asterisk by those that are palpable:

   Lateral epicondyle, femur
   Lateral condyle, femur
   Medial epicondyle, femur
   Medial condyle, femur
   Adductor tubercle
   Patellar surface of femur
   Apex of patella
   Base of patella

   Patellar facet for lateral femoral condyle
   Patellar facet for medial femoral condyle
   Medial condyle of tibia
   Tubercles of intercondylar eminence
   Lateral condyle of tibia
   Head of fibula
   Tibial tuberosity

Figure 4–1

Figure 4–2

Figure 4–3

2. Describe the posterior surface of the patella.

81

3. From an anterior view of a vertical femur, describe the asymmetry of the femoral condyles. What significance does this asymmetry hold for knee posture?

4. In the space below, draw an anterior view and a superior view of the tibial plateau of the left femur including the menisci. Do not include ligaments. Shade the menisci along their areas of attachment.

ARTHROLOGY OF THE KNEE

5. On Figures 4–4 and 4–5, label the following soft tissue structures with the appropriate letter. Draw in the patellar ligament as if it were dissected from the patella but still attached inferiorly.

   a. Medial (tibial) collateral ligament
   b. Lateral (fibular) collateral ligament
   c. Medial meniscus
   d. Lateral meniscus
   e. Anterior cruciate ligament
   f. Posterior cruciate ligament

Figure 4–4

Figure 4–5

*6. On a subject, palpate the following soft tissue structures around the knee.

   Joint line (medial and lateral)
   Medial collateral ligament
   Lateral collateral ligament

   HINT: It is easier to find the joint line if the tibia is passively moved on the femur while you are palpating the area. It is also easier to find the collateral ligaments when you stress the ligament with the joint slightly flexed.

7. List the major articular surfaces and soft tissue structures residing within the articular capsule of the knee. Examine the cruciate ligaments for their relationship to the main articular capsule.

8. The knee is not a pure hinge joint. Why?

*9. The intrajoint actions of spin, roll, and glide are most easily demonstrated in the movements of the knee joint. Examine the chapter on the knee joint in your kinesiology text. Use an anatomical model to demonstrate and explain the following:

   a. How gliding interacts with rolling in knee flexion and extension.

   b. What ligaments guide the femoral condyles in anterior and posterior gliding.

   c. Using the Rule of Three, describe the spinning taking place in the knee during terminal extension in the open and closed kinematic chain situations. What function does this spinning accomplish?

10. What is considered to be full range of motion at the knee? Make sure you give the figures for all of the motions in the knee.

11. Explain the screw-home mechanism including its kinesiological usefulness and the muscle responsible for the unlocking of the knee.

12. In what position of the knee are the medial and lateral collateral ligaments most lax? Taut?

13. In what position of the knee is the anterior cruciate ligament on greatest tension? In what position of the knee is the posterior cruciate ligament on greatest tension?

14. Considering the answers to the ligament tension and screw-home mechanism questions above, what is the close-packed position of the knee? Since rotation of the tibia on the femur is impossible in the close-packed position, you can use this movement to verify your answer.

15. What intrajoint structures occupy sufficient space to keep the joint ligaments taut in extension?

16. Which meniscus is most firmly attached to the tibia and joint capsule?

17. Describe the movement of the medial and lateral menisci as the knee
    a. Extends

    b. Flexes

18. What forces create the meniscal movements described in item 17?

19. Describe the physiological and accessory movements of the patella.

20. Explain (and diagram on Figure 4–6) patellar tracking and the mechanisms by which it is controlled. In your discussion and diagram, include at least:
    a. Vectors representing muscle forces acting on the patella during active extension of the tibia at the knee and the resultant of those forces
    b. Connective tissue support of the patella

c. Bony configuration of the patellofemoral joint

Figure 4-6

*21. For this activity you will need a subject in shorts. Have the subject sit on the edge of a treatment table with feet dangling over the side. Passively extend the right tibia at the knee so the knee is straight. Ask the subject to remain relaxed so there is no active tension in the right quadriceps as you gradually flex the knee. As you flex the knee, passively move the patella medially and laterally at various points in the range of motion.

   a. At what angle of knee flexion are you no longer able to move the patella?

   b. What is the relationship or orientation of the patellar and femoral articular surfaces at that angle?

   c. What will be the primary effect on the patellofemoral joint of an isometric contraction of the quadriceps at that angle?

   d. Passively extend the knee fully and ask for another isometric quadriceps contraction. What is the primary effect on the patellofemoral joint of the isometric contraction in this position?

e. State a principle concerning the effect on the patellofemoral joint of quadriceps contraction at various knee-joint angles.

*22. Measure the Q angle on four subjects. Be sure there is a mix of male and female subjects.
   a. What landmarks did you use to obtain the measurement?

   b. How will an increase in this angle affect patellar tracking?

23. What bursae of the knee are most likely compressed between the floor and the knee when you are kneeling?

MYOLOGY OF THE KNEE

Use the following muscle sheets to aid in learning the origins, insertions, and innervations of the knee muscles. For each of the muscles named, draw in the muscle on the sketch provided and complete the indicated information on the outline.

O: Origin of muscle
I: Insertion of muscle
N: Innervation (both peripheral nerve and spinal level)
R: Relationship of muscle to axis of motion
A: Action of muscle

24. Quadriceps femoris

   Rectus femoris (see description in hip muscles)

   Vastus intermedius
   O: Anterior and lateral surfaces of proximal femoral shaft
   I:
   N: Femoral n. (L-2, L-3, L-4)
   R: Fibers run straight (superior and inferior) from O to I; anterior to axis for flexion and extension
   A: Extension of the tibia at the knee

   Vastus medialis
   O: Distal portion of intertrochanteric line of femur; medial lip of linea aspera; proximal part of medial supracondylar ridge
   I:
   N: Femoral n. (L-2, L-3, L-4)
   R:
   A: Extension of the tibia at the knee

   Vastus lateralis
   O:
   I: Lateral border of patella and then to the tibial tuberosity via the patellar ligament

Figure 4-6

N: Femoral n. (L-2, L-3, L-4)
R:
A: Extension of the tibia at the knee

25. Popliteus
    O:
    I:
    N: Tibial n. (L-4, L-5, S-1)
    R: Fibers run obliquely and inferiorly from O to I; posterior and medial to axis for rotation of tibia at the knee; posterior and lateral to axis for rotation of femur at the knee
    A:

Figure 4-7

26. Plantaris
    O:
    I: Tendocalcaneus
    N:
    R: Fibers run superior and inferior from O to I, in the form of a long, slender tendon; posterior to axes for ankle dorsiflexion and plantarflexion, and for knee flexion and extension
    A: Weak plantarflexion of foot at the ankle; flexion of tibia at the knee

27. Gastrocnemius
    O:
    I: Tendocalcaneus; posterior surface of calcaneus
    N: Tibial n. (S-1, S-2)
    R:
    A: Plantar flexion of the foot at the ankle and flexion of the tibia at the knee

28. Hamstrings [see the chapter on the hip (Chap. 3) for their description]

29. List all the one-joint muscles crossing the knee.

30. List the muscles crossing posterior to the knee joint.

Figure 4-8

APPLICATIONS

*31. Passively flex a subject's knee to 90° and perform passive medial rotation of the tibia at the knee to the end range. The end feel will be firm indicating that the motion is restricted by ligament. Now, passively laterally rotate the tibia. You should find a similar end-feel at the limit of the range of motion. What ligaments are restricting the motion in each case? Note: If you have difficulty figuring out the answer to this question from reading and discussion, try the movements on a cadaver in gross anatomy laboratory, once the knee is dissected and the ligaments can be viewed.

*32. With your subject sitting, muscle test the quadriceps with the subject leaning forward and then leaning back. What difference in muscle strength did you find? Explain the difference.

*33. Determine a position for muscle testing the quadriceps group that allows the greatest tension to be developed by the entire muscle group through the greatest range of motion. Perform the test and compare your results with the standard position for muscle testing the quadriceps. Was there a difference in strength in the two positions? If there was, explain why.

*34. Muscle test the hamstrings with the ankle plantarflexed and then with the ankle dorsiflexed. Did you find a difference in strength in the two positions? Explain your results.

*35. Perform a reasonable test of hamstring strength that requires the muscle to work *against gravity* through the full range of motion. Be sure to allow the muscle to develop maximum tension through maximum range of motion.

*36. Examine the effect on the lumbar spine (in a standing subject) of moving the knees from a normal to a recurvatum position.

*37. Examine the effect on the lumbar spine (in a standing subject) of moving the knees from a normal to a mildly flexed position.

*38. Perform a break test for knee extension with the subject's knee fully extended and then with it flexed 5°. In which position was it easier to break the contraction? Why?

*39. These activities are best done by an individual with normally stable knees.
   a. From an erect standing position, cross the left lower limb in front of the right and place it on the ground, turning to the right while the right foot remains stationary. (The right lower limb will be twisted.)
   What position does the right femur assume in relation to the tibia?

   What knee ligaments are most stressed in this position?

   b. In a normal standing position, what knee ligaments would be most stressed by a sudden valgus stress?

40. Explain the biomechanical and functional implications of a patellectomy. Be sure to include moment arms in your discussion.

41. What muscle group would you strengthen to provide dynamic stability to substitute for the loss of stability of a torn anterior cruciate ligament? Explain your choice.

42. Explain why a positive Apley's compression test with lateral rotation of the tibia on the femur is indicative of a tear in the posterior horn of the medial meniscus. A positive test means that the patient complains of pain during the maneuver.

43. As you move from squatting to standing, the femur extends at the knee producing a rolling of the femoral condyles on the tibial plateau. Explain the intrajoint mechanics which prevent crushing the menisci and anterior dislocation of the femur off the tibia during this movement.

ANSWERS TO KNEE

1. Lateral epicondyle, femur* Patellar facet for lateral femoral condyle
   Lateral condyle, femur* Patellar facet for medial femoral condyle
   Medial epicondyle, femur* Medial condyle of tibia
   Medial condyle, femur* Tubercles of intercondylar eminence
   Adductor tubercle* Lateral condyle of tibia
   Patellar surface of femur Head of fibula*
   Apex of patella* Tibial tuberosity*
   Base of patella*

2. The posterior surface of the patella is multifaceted with a central longitudinal ridge covered with articular cartilage. The central ridge separates the two main articular surfaces, the medial and lateral.

3. The medial condyle projects more distally than the lateral helping to produce the normal valgus in the knee.

4. Check your anatomy text for confirmation of your drawing. In addition to the area of attachment to the coronary ligaments, shade the areas where the transverse ligament joins the two menisci, where the semimembranous muscle and the medial collateral ligament are attached to the medial meniscus, and where the meniscofemoral ligament and popliteus muscle are attached to the lateral meniscus.

5. Check your text and have a faculty member confirm your information.

*6. Have a faculty member confirm your palpations. Deduction of the stress position for each ligament can be made from the structure and function of the ligament. For instance, since the medial collateral ligament resists a valgus stress of the knee and since it is lax in some flexion of the knee, it can be palpated by first relaxing it then placing the knee on a valgus stress.
   Palpating the medial joint line during the valgus maneuver will locate the ligament as it changes from lax to taut. Repeat the problem-solving process for determining the position for palpating the lateral collateral ligament.

7. The joint surfaces within the articular capsule of the knee are the patellar and complimentary femoral surface of the patellofemoral joint, the femoral condyles, and the tibial plateau. The menisci are also within the capsule. The cruciate ligaments reside outside the synovial cavity of the articular capsule, but have independent synovial covering.

8. The knee is not a true hinge joint because it has two degrees of freedom, rotation as well as flexion and extension.

9. a. Gliding maintains the larger joint surface of the femur in contact with the tibia, gliding it forward during flexion of the femur on the tibia, and gliding it back during extension of the femur on the tibia.
   b. The anterior cruciate controls backward roll of the femoral condyles on the tibial plateau during flexion of the femur at the knee. This guides the anterior glide of the femoral condyles on the tibial plateau during flexion of the femur at the knee. The posterior cruciate does the opposite.
   c. In the open kinematic chain, the tibia laterally rotates at the knee at terminal extension. In the closed chain, the femur medially rotates at the knee. This stabilizes the knee when it is in full extension.

10. 135° of active flexion of the tibia at the knee and 40° to 80° of passive rotation of tibia at the knee (depending on author) with the knee at 90° of flexion. About 20° of rotation of the tibia at the knee occur at terminal extension. The figures are the same for the reverse actions.

11. Medial rotation of the femur at the knee (closed kinematic chain), or lateral rotation of the tibia at the knee (open kinematic chain) accomplishes the screw-home mechanism and seats the intercondylar tubercles of the tibia into the intercondylar notch of the femur. It also brings the collateral and cruciate ligaments into their tightest position and seats the femoral condyles tightly into the menisci.

The locked knee position allows standing without active contraction of the antigravity knee muscles. The muscle that unlocks the knee is the popliteus.

12. The medial and lateral collateral ligaments are most lax at 90° of flexion and taut at full extension. They are, of course, also relatively lax between full extension and 90° of flexion, although some portion of the medial collateral ligament is taut throughout the range of flexion and extension.

13. Both cruciates are taut in extension, with the anterior cruciate relatively more so than the posterior. Some fibers of the anterior cruciate are taut throughout the range of motion of flexion and extension. The posterior portion of the posterior cruciate is taut in full flexion while the anterior portion is taut in extension.

14. Full extension is the close-packed position of the knee. The bones are fully congruent and the greatest number of stabilizing ligaments are at their tightest in this position. No rotation is possible in the extended position.

15. The menisci and articular cartilage occupy space and maintain the tension on the ligaments. Loss of these space-occupying tissues causes approximation of the joint surfaces and laxity in the ligaments.

16. The medial meniscus is attached to the medial collateral ligament and the medial capsule. It is more firmly attached to the tibial plateau than the lateral meniscus.

17. a. The menisci slide anteriorly as the knee extends. The lateral meniscus moves further than the medial.
    b. They move posteriorly during flexion.

18. Anterior movement is accomplished by pull from the meniscopatellar ligaments and by the fact that the femoral condyles are rolling anteriorly against the ridges of the menisci. During flexion, they move posteriorly in response to the rolling of the femoral condyles, plus the semitendinosis pulls the medial meniscus posteriorly and the popliteus pulls the lateral meniscus posteriorly by active contraction.

19. The patella is anchored firmly to the tibia by the patellar ligament, so its superior-inferior movement is dependent on movement of the tibia. As the tibia moves into flexion at the knee, it pulls the patella inferiorly in relation to the femur. As the quadriceps pull the tibia into extension at the knee, the patella moves superiorly on the femur.
    In the extended but relaxed position, the patella can be passively moved in medial-lateral and superior-inferior directions.

20. The patella tracks superiorly and inferiorly in the intercondylar groove. Whether it tracks in midline, medially, or laterally depends on the relative forces of the medial and lateral vasti and the patellar retinaculum. The medial and lateral lips of the intercondylar groove of the femur will also tend to guide the movement of the patella. If there is asymmetry in the controlling forces, then it will track to the side with the stronger influence.

*21. a. The angle of flexion when the patella becomes fixed medially and laterally will vary according to individuals.
    b. The patellar articular surfaces are well down the femoral articular surfaces and seated in the interarticular groove. The patella is approaching the distal end of the femur and a position more perpendicular than parallel to the shaft of the femur.
    c. The primary effect will be compression of the patellofemoral joint surfaces.
    d. In full extension, the patella is parallel to the shaft of the femur and contraction of the quadriceps will produce sliding of the patella in the articular groove of the femur, rather than compression against the femur.
    e. With greater flexion of the knee joint, contraction of the quadriceps causes greater compression in the patellofemoral joint. More recent research indicates that the angle of greatest patellofemoral compression may vary depending on whether the knee is in an open or closed kinematic chain.

*22. The normal Q angle varies from 10° to 20°; females normally show a larger angle.
   a. ASIS, midpatella, tibial tuberosity
   b. An increase in the angle will create a bowstring effect since the patella is tethered between the superiorly pulling quadriceps and the inferiorly pulling patellar ligament. The increased Q angle causes greater lateral force on the patella producing greater pressure on the lateral lip of the articular groove of the femur as well as on the lateral articular surface of the patella.

23. The bursae are the prepatellar and infrapatellar.

24. Quadriceps femoris
   a. Rectus femoris (see description in hip muscles)
   b. Vastus intermedius
      O: Anterior and lateral surfaces of proximal femoral shaft
      I: Base of patella and then to the tibial tuberosity via the patellar ligament
      N: Femoral n. (L-2, L-3, L-4)
      R: Fibers run straight (superior and inferior) from O to I; anterior to axis for flexion and extension
      A: Extension of the tibia at the knee
   c. Vastus medialis
      O: Distal portion of intertrochanteric line; medial lip of linea aspera; proximal part of medial supracondylar ridge
      I: Medial border of patella and then to the tibial tuberosity via the patellar ligament
      N: Femoral n. (L-2, L-3, L-4)
      R: Fibers run straight (superior and inferior) from O to I; anterior to axis for flexion and extension (most medial of quadriceps and therefore pulls the patella medially)
      A: Extension of the tibia at the knee
   d. Vastus lateralis
      O: Anterior portion of greater trochanter; proximal portion of intertrochanteric line; proximal half of lateral lip of linea aspera
      I: Lateral border of patella and then to the tibial tuberosity via the patellar ligament
      N: Femoral n. (L-2, L-3, L-4)
      R: Fibers run straight (superior and inferior) from O to I; anterior to axis for flexion and extension (most lateral of the quadriceps and therefore pulls the patella laterally)
      A: Extension of the tibia at the knee

25. Popliteus
   O: Posterior surface of lateral epicondyle of femur
   I: Posterior surface of medial proximal tibia
   N: Tibial n. (L-4, L-5, S-1)
   R: Fibers run obliquely and inferiorly from O to I; posterior and medial to axis for rotation of tibia at the knee; posterior and lateral to axis for rotation of femur at the knee
   A: Medial rotation of tibia at the knee (open kinematic chain); lateral rotation of the femur at the knee (closed kinematic chain)

26. Plantaris
   O: Posterior surface of lateral epicondyle of femur
   I: Tendocalcaneus
   N: Tibial n. (L-5, S-1)
   R: Fibers run superior and inferior from O to I, in the form of a long, slender tendon; posterior to axes for ankle dorsiflexion and plantarflexion, and for knee flexion and extension
   A: Weak plantarflexion of foot at the ankle; flexion of tibia at the knee

27. Gastrocnemius
    O: Posterior surface of medial and lateral epicondyles of femur
    I: Tendocalcaneus; posterior surface of calcaneus
    N: Tibial n. (S-1, S-2)
    R: From each origin to midline of muscle to form two heads; posterior to axis for knee flexion and extension; posterior to axis for ankle plantarflexion and dorsiflexion
    A: Plantar flexion of the foot at the ankle; flexion of the tibia at the knee

28. Hamstrings [see the chapter on the hip (Chap. 3)]

29. The one-joint muscles crossing the knee are the

    Biceps short head
    Popliteus
    Vastus lateralis
    Vastus intermedius
    Vastus medialis

30. The muscles crossing posterior to the knee are the

    Hamstrings
    Popliteus
    Gastrocnemius
    Plantaris

*31. This activity reinforces the sensation of a ligamentous end-feel and can lead into the mechanics of knee ligament injuries. The firm end-feel at the end-range of medial rotation of the tibia on the femur is the result of tightening of the anterior and posterior cruciate ligaments; in lateral rotation it is of the medial and lateral collateral ligaments.

*32. This activity demonstrates a functional relevance of active insufficiency and body position during exercise or muscle testing. It also can lead to discussion of the relative contribution of the rectus femoris to the force of the quadriceps, and the effect of hip position on that force.

*33. There are several possible solutions to this problem. However, each must satisfy the criterion of preventing active insufficiency in the rectus as the knee approaches full extension.

*34. This is another length-tension relationship problem, demonstrating how a muscle with primary function at the ankle (gastrocnemius) can affect the force of flexion of the tibia at the knee. The learners will most likely find that knee flexion is stronger with the ankle dorsiflexed than with it plantarflexed. This can lead to the rationalization of the hamstring muscle-testing position with the ankle plantarflexed.

*35. Again, there are many possible solutions, but they must all position the limb so that flexion of the tibia is never assisted by gravity and must allow hip motion to compensate for the hamstring muscle shortening over the knee. An example could be to position the subject in a standing position and have her simultaneously flex her hip and knee.

*36. Genu recurvatum produces a compensatory increase in lumbar lordosis.

*37. Standing with knee flexion produces a compensatory decrease in the lumbar lordosis.

*38. The learners should find it easier to break the isometric contraction with the knee slightly flexed because the fully extended knee is locked and has ligamentous stability, while the partially flexed knee relies mainly on muscle strength to maintain the position.

*39. a. Lateral rotation; cruciates
     b. Medial collateral; anterior cruciate

40. Removal of the patella removes the pulley effect for the quadriceps over the knee, thus bringing the line of pull of the muscle closer to the axis of motion. This change in line of pull of the quadriceps decreases the moment arm of the muscle force, thus diminishing the effective strength of the muscle. Patellectomy functionally weakens the quadriceps.

41. The hamstrings because their line of pull puts a posterior translatory force on the tibia, pulling it posteriorly on the femur as well as rotating the tibia into flexion.

42. The meniscus is compressed as the tibia is pressed downward onto the condyle of the femur. Lateral rotation of the tibia asymmetrically stresses the posterior horn of the medial meniscus.

43. The condyles of the femur glide posteriorly as the knee extends because of the tethering provided by the posterior cruciate ligament. This keeps the articular surfaces in contact and the femur on the tibia. The rolling of the femoral condyles and the pull of the meniscopatellar ligaments bring the menisci forward avoiding their compression between the condyles and the tibial plateau.

CHAPTER 5

Foot and Ankle

OSTEOLOGY OF THE FOOT AND ANKLE

The Foot

1. On Figures 5-1, 5-2, and 5-3, identify and label the bones listed below. Familiarize yourself with these bones and landmarks by identifying them in text drawings and on a skeleton.

    Phalanges
    Metatarsals
    Tubercle of metatarsals
    Tuberosity of fifth metatarsal
    Cuneiforms
    Cuboid
    Tuberosity of cuboid
    Talus (head and neck)
    Calcaneus
    Sustentaculum tali
    Peroneal tubercle of calcaneus
    Navicular tubercle

Figure 5-1

Figure 5-2

Figure 5-3

2. What is the function of the sustentaculum tali of the calcaneus?

3. What is the function of the navicular tuberosity?

The Ankle

*4. Familiarize yourself with the structures listed below by identifying them on the skeleton and then palpating them on yourself and a classmate.

   Medial malleolus
   Lateral malleolus
   Distal portion of shaft of tibia
   Distal portion of shaft of fibula
   Joint line of talocrural joint

5. What is the function of the sulcus tali of the talus?

6. Define tibial torsion. How does normal tibial torsion affect the foot in stance? What is the normal amount of tibial torsion evident during stance?

7. Define external or lateral and internal or medial tibial torsion.

ARTHROLOGY OF THE FOOT AND ANKLE

8. Complete the outline below:

   Superior tibiofibular joint
       Type of joint

       Bones involved

       Movement(s) permitted

   Inferior tibiofibular joint
       Type of joint

       Bones involved

       Movement(s) permitted

Talocrural joint
    Type of joint

    Bones involved

    Movement(s) permitted

Subtalar joint (talocalcaneal joint)
    Type of joint

    Bones involved

    Movement(s) permitted

Talocalcaneonavicular joint
    Type of joint

    Bones involved

    Movement(s) permitted

Calcaneocuboid joint
    Type of joint

    Bones involved

    Movement(s) permitted

Talonavicular joint
    Type of joint

    Bones involved

    Movement(s) permitted

Tarsometatarsal joints
    Type of joint

    Bones involved

    Movement(s) permitted

Metatarsophalangeal joints
    Type of joint

    Bones involved

    Movement(s) permitted

Interphalangeal joints
    Type of joint

    Bones involved

    Movement(s) permitted

*9. With your laboratory partner sitting on a treatment table with her legs extended, hold the distal end of her tibia firmly. With your other hand, try to move the distal end of the fibula posteriorly (down toward the table). What, if any, motion do you feel? What limits motion at the inferior tibiofibular joint?

10. Why is the talocrural joint referred to as a mortise and tenon joint?

11. In view of the shape of the articular surface of the talus, what motion is required of the mortise during dorsiflexion? Hint: look at the shape of the articular surface of the talus.

*12. Passively take your partner's foot into full eversion and full inversion. In which direction were you able to obtain more motion? What is the relationship of your finding to the asymmetry between the medial and lateral malleoli?

13. Define the following terms as they apply to movements of the foot and ankle. (some of them appear in Chap. 1). Go to several sources for your definitions. You will probably note that different sources use the same terms to mean different motions. It will be important for you to be aware of all of the definitions so that you can communicate accurately about ankle motions.

    Dorsiflexion:

    Plantarflexion:

    Inversion:

    Eversion:

    Pronation:

    Supination:

    Abduction:

    Adduction:

14. Which foot and ankle joints allow inversion with supination (making the soles of the feet face each other) and eversion with pronation (making the soles of the feet face away from each other)? If you wanted to surgically eliminate these motions, what joints would you need to fuse?

15. In which position is the transverse tarsal joint close packed?

16. In which position is the transverse tarsal joint open packed?

17. Which of the tarsometatarsal joints share a joint capsule?

18. What is the function of the metatarsophalangeal joint in the weight-bearing foot?

19. What is the function of the interphalangeal joints of the toes in the weight-bearing foot?

20. What is the primary function of the ligaments of the ankle-foot complex? Why do we attend to these ligaments in more detail than with some other joints?

21. a. What is the specific function of the anterior tibiofibular, posterior tibiofibular, and crural interosseous tibiofibular ligaments?

    b. Draw the two tibiofibular ligaments on Figures 5–2 and 5–3 and label them.

Figure 5–2

Figure 5–3

*22. a. What is the specific function of the anterior talofibular, posterior talofibular, calcaneofibular, long plantar, and short plantar ligaments?

b. Draw and label each ligament on Figure 5–2 in item 21.
c. Passively stress each of the ligaments.
d. Palpate each of the ligaments that are palpable.

23. In an inversion-plantarflexion injury, which ligaments are most likely to be injured?

24. Which of the lateral ligaments is the weakest?

*25. a. What is the function of the deltoid ligament and the spring ligament?

b. Draw the four parts of the deltoid ligament and the spring ligament on Figure 5–3. Label the parts of the deltoid ligament.

Figure 5–3

c. Stress the deltoid and the spring ligaments.
d. Palpate the deltoid ligament.
e. Palpate the calcaneal attachment of the spring ligament.

26. a. High stress in what position could cause disruption of the deltoid ligament?

b. Is disruption of this ligament likely?

c. Why or why not?

27. What are the attachments and function of the deep transverse metatarsal ligament?

ARCHES OF THE FOOT

28. Complete the following outline:
    Medial longitudinal arch
        Bones involved:

        Major support:

    Lateral longitudinal arch
        Bones involved:

        Major support:

    Transverse arch
        Bones involved:

        Major support:

*29. Examine someone for flat feet. A normal medial longitudinal arch measures 15 to 18 mm from the ground to the navicular tubercle. What anatomical structures are responsible for maintaining this arch?

*30. What other major joint(s) of the body would be affected by pathological pronation of the foot in stance? How would they be affected? Demonstrate your explanation with an articulated skeleton of a knee, foot, and ankle.

MYOLOGY OF THE FOOT AND ANKLE

Use the following muscle sheets to aid in learning the origins, insertions, and innervations of the foot muscles. For each muscle named, draw in the muscle on the sketch and complete the indicated information on the outline. The following abbreviations apply throughout the muscle sheets:
- O: Origin of muscle
- I: Insertion of muscle
- N: Innervation (both spinal level and peripheral nerve)
- R: Relationship of muscle to axis of motion
- A: Action of muscle

31. Tibialis posterior
    O: Medial surface of proximal two thirds of fibula; interosseous membrane; posterolateral surface of tibia
    I: Tuberosity of navicular; plantar surfaces of sustentaculum of calcaneus; three cuneiforms; cuboid; bases of second, third, and fourth metatarsals (does not attach to talus posteriorly or to first and fifth metatarsal anteriorly)
    N: Tibial n. (L-5, S-1)
    R: Courses straight and slightly anteriorly; winds around posterior surface of medial malleolus; enters the sole of the foot; winds around talus and then divides into its numerous insertions; medial to axis for inversion and eversion
    A:

32. Peroneus longus
    O: Superior two thirds of lateral surface of fibula
    I: Lateral aspect of base of first metatarsal and medial cuneiform
    N: Superficial peroneal n. (L-4, L-5, S-1)
    R: Tendon courses inferiorly and winds around posterior aspect of lateral malleolus; continues in a groove on plantar surface of cuboid; crosses plantar surface of foot to reach insertion; lateral to axis for inversion and eversion; slightly posterior to axis for dorsiflexion and plantarflexion
    A:

33. Peroneus brevis
    O:
    I:
    N:
    R:
    A:

Figure 5-4

34. Tibialis anterior
    O:
    I:
    N:
    R:
    A:

35. Extensor digitorum longus
    O:
    I:
    N:
    R:
    A:

Figure 5–5

36. Extensor digitorum brevis
    O:
    I:
    N:
    R:
    A:

37. Extensor hallucis longus
    O:
    I:
    N:
    R:
    A:

Figure 5–5

38. Gastrocnemius
    O:
    I:
    N:
    R:
    A:

39. Soleus
    O:
    I:
    N:
    R:
    A:

40. Plantaris
    O:
    I:
    N:
    R:
    A:

Figure 5-6

41. Flexor digitorum brevis

    O: Calcaneus
    I: Middle phalanges of lateral four toes
    N: Medial plantar n. (L-4, L-5)
    R:
    A:

42. Abductor hallucis

    O:
    I:
    N:
    R:
    A:

Figure 5–7

43. Flexor hallucis longus

    O: Lower two thirds of posterior fibula
    I: Base of distal phalanx of great toe
    N: Tibial n. (L-5, S-1, S-2)
    R: Plantar to axis for flexion and extension; posterior to axis for dorsiflexion and plantarflexion
    A:

44. Flexor digitorum longus

    O:
    I:
    N:
    R:
    A:

45. Peroneus longus tendon (see item 32)

46. Tibialis posterior tendon (see item 31)

Figure 5–4

APPLICATIONS

*47. Test the strength of the gastrocnemius with the knee fully flexed and with the knee extended. Note the difference in strength of contraction of the gastrocnemius with the knee flexed versus with the knee extended. What principle does this illustrate? What are the implications of this for manual muscle testing?

*48. Place your partner's limb in the most effective position to lengthen (stretch) the gastrocnemius muscle. Explain.

*49. Demonstrate an isolated contraction of each of the muscles listed below. What instructions would be helpful to a patient to accomplish these isolated contractions? Be able to palpate each tendon.
   a. Tibialis anterior
   b. Extensor hallucis longus
   c. Extensor digitorum longus

50. Explain why strengthening the peroneus longus and brevis is important following an inversion sprain of the ankle.

*51. In small groups, work with an articulated skeleton of the foot and ankle. Complete and discuss the following motions.
   a. In an open kinematic chain, laterally rotate the tibia on the femur. In what position does this place the foot? How does lateral rotation of the tibia reorient the axis of the ankle joint?

   b. In an open kinematic chain, medially rotate the tibia on the femur. In what position does this place the foot? How does medial rotation of the tibia reorient the axis of the ankle joint?

   c. In a closed kinematic chain, laterally rotate the tibia on the femur. In what position does this place the foot? What other joints of the foot are affected by lateral rotation of the tibia? What other joints of the body might be affected by long-term lateral tibial rotation?

   d. In a closed kinematic chain, medially rotate the tibia on the femur. In what position does this place the foot? What other joints of the foot are affected by medial rotation of the tibia?

*52. Using a skeleton, move the calcaneus on the talus. What intrajoint motion occurs between these two bones? What classical motion does this allow?

*53. On a laboratory partner, palpate the following structures:

First metatarsocuneiform joint	Lateral malleolus
Navicular tubercle	Metatarsal heads
Medial malleolus	Dorsal pedal pulse
Fifth metatarsal bone	Tibialis posterior tendon to insertion
Fifth metatarsophalangeal joint	Peroneus brevis tendon to insertion
Calcaneus	Peroneus tertius
Sustentaculum tali	Tibialis anterior tendon
Peroneal tubercle	Extensor hallucis longus tendon

*54. On your partner, put a dot over the base of the fifth metatarsal and another dot over the head of the fifth metatarsal. Have your partner sit on a treatment table with the knee flexed and the foot over the edge. Position the foot so that the sole of the foot is parallel to the floor. Are the two dots in a line parallel to the floor? What are the implications of this for goniometry of the ankle?

*55. Measure at least five classmates for tibial torsion (amount of toe-out with the tibia facing directly forward); you can measure this with a goniometer. What variation between individuals did you find? Were any of these individuals considered abnormal?

*56. Measure ankle dorsiflexion with the knee extended, then with the knee flexed. Did you find a difference in measurement between the two positions? If you did, explain why you did.

ANSWERS TO FOOT AND ANKLE

1. Check your text and confirm your information with a faculty member.

2. The shelflike projection of the calcaneus known as the sustentaculum tali articulates with and supports the talus and serves as attachment for the spring ligament.

3. Attachment for the tibialis posterior.

*4. Check with your text and confirm your information with a faculty member.

5. The deep groove of the talus, the sulcus tali, serves as the attachment for the interosseous ligament.

6. The torsion or twisting of the distal tibia laterally as compared to the proximal portion is called tibial torsion. This produces a toe-out position of the foot in relation to the leg of 20° to 30°.

7. External or lateral tibial torsion is a pathological increase in tibial torsion. Internal or medial tibial torsion is the pathological decrease in tibial torsion.

8. Superior tibiofibular joint
      Type of joint: plane, synovial joint
      Bones involved: fibula and tibia
      Movements permitted: slight superior and inferior sliding of the fibula and fibular rotation
   Inferior tibiofibular joint
      Type of joint: syndesmosis
      Bones involved: tibia and fibula
      Movements permitted: slight separation and gliding
   Talocrural joint
      Type of joint: hinge, synovial joint
      Bones involved: talus, tibia, and fibula
      Movements permitted: dorsiflexion and plantarflexion
   Subtalar (talocalcaneal) joint
      Type of joint: plane, synovial joint
      Bones involved: talus and calcaneus
      Movements permitted: inversion and eversion
   Talocalcaneonavicular joint
      Type of joint: plane, synovial joint
      Bones involved: talus, navicular, and calcaneus
      Movements permitted: eversion and inversion
   Calcaneocuboid joint
      Type of joint: plane, synovial joint
      Bones involved: calcaneus and cuboid
      Movements permitted: inversion and eversion
   Talonavicular joint
      Type of joint: plane, synovial joint
      Bones involved: talus and navicular
      Movements permitted: inversion and eversion
   Tarsometatarsal joints
      Type of joint: plane, synovial joint
      Bones involved: distal tarsal row and metatarsals
      Movements permitted: inversion and eversion
   Metatarsophalangeal joints
      Type of joint: condyloid, synovial joint
      Bones involved: metatarsals and phalanges
      Movements permitted: extension, flexion, abduction, and adduction
   Interphalangeal joints
      Type of joint: hinge, synovial joint
      Bones involved: phalanges
      Movements permitted: flexion and extension

*9. Some motion is available in this direction. It is limited by fibroadipose tissue and interosseous ligament.

10. The tibia and fibula form an almost-rectangular concave articular surface for the almost-rectangular convex talar head to articulate with. This resembles a mortise and tenon joint in carpentry.

11. The trochlea rotates posteriorly in the ankle mortise with dorsiflexion. The malleoli tend to separate because the superior articular surface of the talus is wider anteriorly than posteriorly.

*12. You were probably able to obtain more inversion than eversion. The more distal position of the lateral malleolus serves to limit the motion of the ankle in eversion. Functionally, this increases the stability of the ankle.

13. Use your texts to confirm your answers.

14. Eversion is a combination of abduction, pronation, and dorsiflexion at the ankle joint. Inversion is a combination of adduction, supination, and plantarflexion at the ankle joint. The talocalcaneonavicular, talonavicular, and subtalar joints allow inversion with supination (or eversion with pronation). To eliminate the motion all three joints would have to be fused.

15. The transverse tarsal joint is close packed in inversion.

16. The transverse tarsal joint is open packed in eversion.

17. The second and third tarsometatarsal joints share a joint capsule. The fourth and fifth tarsometatarsal joints share a joint capsule. Gliding or sliding motions occur at these joints.

18. The metatarsophalangeal joints allow the rigid inverted foot to pass over the weight-bearing toes.

19. The interphalangeal joints help maintain stability by pressing into the ground in static posture and during ambulation as needed. Weight is shifted to the opposite foot in gait by the toes.

20. Static stabilization. The ankle ligaments are commonly injured; therefore, their position and function need to be well understood.

21. a. Maintaining a stable mortise.
    b. Check your text to confirm your information.

*22. a. The anterior talofibular, posterior talofibular, and calcaneofibular ligaments limit distraction of the talus from the fibula (this might occur in severe inversion). The long and short plantar ligaments help maintain the longitudinal arches of the foot.
    b. Check your text to confirm your information.
    c. and d. Have your instructor confirm your accuracy.

23. Anterior talofibular, posterior talofibular, and calcaneofibular ligaments

24. The anterior talofibular ligament

*25. a. The deltoid ligament is designed to control distraction of the talus and tibia and hold the calcaneus and navicular against the talus. The spring ligament assists in maintaining the medial longitudinal arch of the foot.
    b. Check your text to confirm your information.
    c, d, and e. Have your instructor confirm your accuracy.

26. a. Eversion
    b. No
    c. Because of the strength of the ligament, fracture of the malleolus rather than tearing of the ligament is more likely.

27. The attachments are the heads of the metatarsals and the ligament helps maintain the transverse arch of the foot.

28. Medial longitudinal arch
    Bones involved: talus, calcaneus, navicular, three cuneiforms, and three metatarsal bones
    Major support: spring (plantar calcaneonavicular) ligament
    Lateral longitudinal arch
    Bones involved: calcaneus, cuboid, and the lateral two metatarsals
    Major support: long plantar ligament, short plantar ligament, and plantar aponeurosis
    Transverse arch
    Bones involved: cuboid, three cuneiforms, and metatarsals
    Major support: bony structure, the peroneus longus muscle, and deep transverse metatarsal ligament

*29. Use this exercise to gain an appreciation for the range of normal, and perhaps to see some abnormal arches of the feet. The ligamentous structures responsible for maintaining the medial longitudinal arch are the long and short plantar ligaments, the spring ligament, and the plantar aponeurosis. In addition to ligamentous support, the bones themselves help support the arches. Muscles contribute relatively little to the support of the arches.

*30. With severe pes planus, the navicular and the head of the talus come in contact with the ground. The heel and forefoot are everted. This causes genu valgus. Over a prolonged period of time, this pathology may lead to hip degeneration and low back problems because of the prolonged application of abnormal forces through the knees.

31. Tibialis posterior
    O: Medial surface of proximal two thirds of fibula; interosseous membrane; posterolateral surface of tibia
    I: Tuberosity of navicular; plantar surfaces of sustentaculum of calcaneus; cuneiforms; cuboid; bases of second, third, and fourth metatarsals
    N: Tibial n. (L-5, S-1)
    R: Medial to axis for inversion and eversion; posterior to axis for plantarflexion
    A: Plantarflexion, inversion

32. Peroneus longus
    O: Proximal two thirds of lateral surface of fibula
    I: Lateral aspect of base of first metatarsal and medial cuneiform
    N: Superficial peroneal n. (L-4, L-5, S-1)
    R: Lateral to axis for inversion and eversion; posterior to axis for dorsiflexion and plantarflexion
    A: Eversion and plantarflexion

33. Peroneus brevis
    O: Distal two thirds of lateral surface of fibula
    I: Lateral aspect of base of fifth metatarsal
    N: Superficial peroneal n. (L-4, L-5, S-1)
    R: Lateral to axis for inversion and eversion; posterior to axis for dorsiflexion and plantarflexion
    A: Eversion and plantarflexion

34. Tibialis anterior
    O: Superior two thirds of lateral surface of tibia
    I: Medial surface of first cuneiform; base of first metatarsal
    N: Deep peroneal n. (L-4, L-5, S-1)
    R: Anterior to axis for dorsiflexion and plantarflexion; medial to axis for inversion and eversion
    A: Dorsiflexion and inversion

35. Extensor digitorum longus
    O: Superior three quarters of anterior surface of fibula and lateral condyle of tibia
    I: Divides into four tendons which insert onto the middle and distal phalanges of the lateral four digits
    N: Deep peroneal n. (L-4, L-5, S-1)
    R: Anterior to axis for flexion and extension; anterior to axis for ankle dorsiflexion and plantarflexion
    A: Extension of lateral four toes and ankle dorsiflexion

36. Extensor digitorum brevis
    O: Dorsal surface of calcaneus
    I: Divides into four tendons which insert into the proximal phalanx of great toe and tendons of extensor digitorum longus of the second, third, and fourth toes
    N: Deep peroneal n. (L-5, S-1)
    R: Anterior to axis for flexion and extension
    A: Extension of medial four toes

37. Extensor hallucis longus
    O: Middle third of anterior surface of fibula
    I: Base of distal phalanx of great toe
    N: Deep peroneal n. (L-4, L-5, S-1)
    R: Dorsal to axis for extension and flexion; anterior to axis for dorsiflexion and plantarflexion of foot
    A: Extension of great toe and dorsiflexion of ankle

38. Gastrocnemius
    O: Medial head: proximal and posterior aspect of medial condyle of femur
       Lateral head: lateral condyle of femur
    I: Tendocalcaneus which attaches to proximal posterior surface of calcaneus
    N: Tibial n. (S-1, S-2)
    R: Posterior to the axes for ankle plantarflexion and dorsiflexion and knee flexion and extension
    A: Plantarflexion of ankle

39. Soleus
    O: Posterior surface of head and shaft of fibula and body; middle third of medial tibia
    I: Tendocalcaneus (see gastrocnemius)
    N: Tibial n. (S-1, S-2)
    R: Posterior to the axis for plantarflexion and dorsiflexion of the ankle
    A: Plantarflexion of ankle

40. Plantaris
    O: Distal part of supracondylar line of femur
    I: Tendocalcaneus (see gastrocnemius)
    N: Tibial n. (S-1, S-2)
    R: Posterior to the axis for ankle plantarflexion and dorsiflexion
    A: Plantarflexion

41. Flexor digitorum brevis
    O: Calcaneus
    I: Middle phalanges of lateral four toes
    N: Medial plantar n. (L-4, L-5)
    R: Plantar to axis for flexion and extension
    A: Flexion of lateral four toes

42. Abductor hallucis
    O: Flexor retinaculum and calcaneus
    I: Base of proximal phalanx of great toe
    N: Medial plantar n. (S-2, S-3)
    R: Lateral and proximal to the axis for great toe abduction and adduction
    A: Abduction of great toe

43. Flexor hallucis longus
    O: Lower two thirds of posterior fibula
    I: Base of distal phalanx of great toe
    N: Tibial n. (L-5, S-1, S-2)
    R: Plantar to axis for flexion and extension
    A: Flexion of great toe

44. Flexor digitorum longus
    O: Posterior aspect of tibia
    I: Four tendons insert on the distal phalanges of lateral four digits
    N: Tibial n. (L-5, S-1)
    R: Posterior to axis for plantarflexion and dorsiflexion; plantar to axis for flexion and extension of the toes.
    A: Flexion of lateral four toes and plantarflexion of ankle

FOOT AND ANKLE ■ 113

45. See item 32, above.

46. See item 31, above.

47. With the knee flexed and the foot plantarflexed, the gastrocnemius generates less force (is weaker) due to active insufficiency. This, therefore, could provide a good position for ruling out the gastrocnemius when you want to assess the strength of the soleus.

48. The gastrocnemius can be stretched effectively by simultaneously causing knee extension and ankle dorsiflexion.

49. a. Helpful instructions for getting an isolated contraction of the tibialis anterior might be to give the subject a goal to touch (your hand, for instance) as you say, "Touch my hand with your big toe."
    b. Helpful instructions for getting an isolated contraction of the extensor hallucis longus might be "Let your foot hang loosely while you try gently to raise your big toe. Do not raise your other toes."
    c. Helpful instructions for getting an isolated contraction of the extensor digitorum longus might be "Let your foot hang loosely while you try gently to raise your toes without raising your big toe."
    NOTE: To get an isolated contraction, you may need to instruct your subject to try *gently* or *easily* so that he does not activate any muscles other than the one you are after.

50. With inversion sprains of the ankle, the peroneal muscles are stretched. This overstretching may cause weakening of the muscles. Strengthening these muscles may also help prevent reinjury to the area by strengthening the muscles that would resist inversion.

*51. a. This puts the foot in a toe-out position. Normal tibial torsion rotates the axis of the ankle joint to a line that is anterior medially and posterior laterally; by externally rotating the tibia further, this position is accentuated.
    b. This puts the foot in a neutral or toe-in position. This puts the axis in a plane closer to the frontal plane than the previous activity.
    c. The foot remains in the same position in relation to the supporting surface in which it started. In relation to the tibia, though, the foot is now more in a position of toe-in. The other joints of the foot will adjust to allow the sole of the foot to maintain contact with the floor. The medial longitudinal arch will be elevated. The knee and hip will also be affected by this rotation of the tibia.
    d. The foot remains in the same position in relation to the supporting surface in which it started. In relation to the tibia, though, the foot is now more in a position of toe-out. The other joints of the foot will adjust to allow the sole of the foot to maintain contact with the floor. This position will tend to depress the medial longitudinal arch. The knee and hip will also be affected by this rotation of the tibia.

*52. Gliding occurs and results in inversion and eversion.

*53. Check with a text and confirm your information with a faculty member.

*54. The fifth metatarsal and the sole of the foot are not parallel. Therefore, if the sole of the foot is parallel to the floor, the fifth metatarsal cannot be. The implication for goniometry is that the two different referrents cannot be used interchangeably. Either reference (head and base of fifth metatarsal or sole of foot) can be used, but different readings will be obtained.

*55. Use this activity to explore the range of normal.

*56. In most individuals you will find increased dorsiflexion with knee flexion. By flexing the knee, the gastrocnemius is put on slack and will not limit dorsiflexion. When the knee is extended and the ankle dorsiflexed, the gastrocnemius may be passively insufficient.

CHAPTER 6

Shoulder

OSTEOLOGY OF THE SHOULDER

The shoulder complex allows great mobility in the upper extremity, but at the expense of stability. Its articulations are loose allowing the bones a wide range of motion.

1. What are the bones of the shoulder complex? (Ignore the ribs for now.)

*2. Identify the following landmarks on a skeleton, then palpate as many of them as possible on a partner. Locate all of them on Figures 6–1, 6–2, and 6–3.

Scapula

Inferior angle
Superior angle
Medial border
Lateral border
Coracoid process
Spine
Acromion
Glenoid fossa
Infraglenoid tubercle
Supraglenoid tubercle

Clavicle

Sternal end
Anterior concavity
Acromial end

Humerus

Head
Anatomical neck
Surgical neck
Greater tubercle
Lesser tubercle
Bicipital groove
Deltoid tuberosity

Sternum

Sternal notch
Xyphoid process

Figure 6-1

Figure 6-2

Figure 6-3

3. Describe the orientation of the surface of the glenoid fossa in relationship to the trunk when the shoulder girdle is in the normal resting position. You may need an accurately articulated skeleton to answer this question.

4. Discuss the relative congruence of the humeral head and glenoid fossa. Hint: look at the size and shape of each. In your discussion, include the relationship of congruence to stability of the glenohumeral joint.

ARTHROLOGY OF THE SHOULDER

The articulations of the shoulder complex are:

Diarthrodial joints:
    Sternoclavicular
    Acromioclavicular
    Glenohumeral
Functional joints:
    Scapulothoracic
    Coracoacromial arch

Fill in the necessary information about the joints and articulations in the outline and diagrams below.

Sternoclavicular Joint:

5. Give the type of diarthrodial joint, number of degrees of freedom of movement, and movements available at the sternoclavicular joint. How are the names of the movements determined?

6. Label each of the following ligaments on Figure 6–4:
   Interclavicular ligament
   Costoclavicular ligament
   Anterior and posterior sternoclavicular ligaments

Figure 6–4

7. Give a description and discuss the role of the articular disc of the sternoclavicular (SC) joint.

8. Give the function (control of motion or stabilization) of each of the ligaments associated with the sternoclavicular joint.

   a. Interclavicular

   b. Costoclavicular

   c. Anterior and posterior sternoclavicular

*9. Perform the following clavicular motions yourself, then observe them on a partner. Beside each motion, note what extremity or scapular motion was required to produce the clavicular motion.
   a. Elevation: _____
   b. Depression: _____
   c. Protraction: _____
   d. Retraction: _____
   e. Rotation: _____

Acromioclavicular Joint

10. Give the type of joint and number of degrees of freedom of movement at the acromioclavicular joint. In your own words, give the motions of the scapula at the acromioclavicular joint.

11. Label each of the following ligaments on Figure 6–5:
    Coracoclavicular ligament
    Acromioclavicular ligament
    Coracoacromial ligament

Figure 6–5

12. Give the function (control of motion or stabilization) of each of the liagaments associated with the acromioclavicular joint.
    a. Coracoclavicular
       Conoid portion
       Trapezoid portion

    b. Acromioclavicular

    c. Coracoacromial

Glenohumeral Joint

13. Give the type of joint and number of degrees of freedom of the glenohumeral joint.

14. On Figure 6–5 in item 11, label the following ligaments of the glenohumeral joint:
    Glenohumeral ligament
    Coracohumeral ligament

*15. Select a subject with her back exposed. Stabilize the right scapula with your right hand on the lateral border so that it does not move laterally during abduction or flexion of the humerus at the shoulder. Ask the subject to flex the humerus at the shoulder. Make sure the scapula does not move. Then ask her to abduct the humerus at the shoulder. Again, make sure the scapula does not move. Now, repeat the motions and allow the scapula to participate in each of the movements freely.
   Now, press your hand on the flat of the scapula so that the inferior angle of the scapula maintains close contact with the chest wall. Ask the subject to rotate the humerus medially at the shoulder with the scapula stabilized and then with it free to move.
   Describe the difference in range of motion available in all of these situations.

16. Describe the movement of the humeral head on the glenoid fossa during abduction of the humerus at the shoulder.

17. During abduction of the humerus, what force keeps the humeral head from rolling superiorly off the glenoid fossa?

18. Describe the major bursa of the shoulder joint associated with abduction of the humerus at the shoulder and give its main functions.

19. Give the attachments for the joint capsule of the glenohumeral joint. Describe the capsule's outstanding features and the functional implications of those features.

Scapulothoracic Joint

20. Name the motions of the scapula, giving all the synonyms for the motions that occur in various readings such as your kinesiology text, muscle testing text, anatomy text, and goniometry text.

21. Describe, in your own words, scapulohumeral rhythm.

22. Which of the joints of the shoulder girdle is the only bony attachment of the shoulder girdle to the trunk?

MYOLOGY OF THE SHOULDER

Use the following muscle sheets to aid in learning the origins, insertions, and innervations of the shoulder muscles. For each of the muscles named, draw in the muscle on the sketch and complete the indicated information in the outline.

    O: Origin of muscle
    I: Insertion of muscle
    N: Innervation (both peripheral nerve and spinal level)
    R: Relationship of muscle to axis of motion
    A: Action of muscle

23. Pectoralis major
    O: Anterior surface of clavicle, sternum
    I: Greater tubercle of humerus
    N: Medial and lateral pectoral n. s (C-5, C-6, C-7, C-8, T-1)
    R: Fibers run obliquely and horizontally; medial (or inferior) to axis for abduction and adduction; anterior and wraps around longitudinally to axis for medial rotation; medial to axis for horizontal abduction and adduction
    A: Adduction, horizontal adduction, and medial rotation of the humerus at the shoulder

24. Pectoralis minor
    O:
    I:
    N: Medial pectoral n. (C-6, C-7, C-8, T-1)
    R: Fibers run upward and obliquely from medial to lateral
    A: Downward scapular rotation and anterior tipping of the scapula

25. Serratus anterior
    O: Outer superior border of 1st 8–9 ribs
    I:
    N:
    R: Line of force runs from anterior on the thorax to posterior on the medial border of the scapula
    A: Scapular abduction (protraction); some upward rotation of scapula

26. Coracobrachialis
    O: Coracoid process
    I: Middle third of the medial surface of the shaft of the humerus
    N: Musculocutaneous n. (C-6, C-7)
    R:
    A: Shoulder flexion and slight adduction

Figure 6–6

Figure 6–6

27. Supraspinatus
    O: Supraspinous fossa of the scapula
    I:
    N: Suprascapular n. (C-4, C-5, C-6)
    R:
    A: Abduction of the humerus at the shoulder; compresses humeral head onto the glenoid fossa

28. Teres minor
    O:
    I: Lowest point of greater tubercle of humerus
    N:
    R: Obliquely upward from O to I; wraps around longitudinal axis posterolaterally
    A: Lateral rotation of the humerus at the shoulder

29. Infraspinatus
    O:
    I: Middle point of greater tubercle of humerus
    N: Suprascapular n. (C-4, C-5, C-6)
    R:
    A: Lateral rotation of the humerus at the shoulder

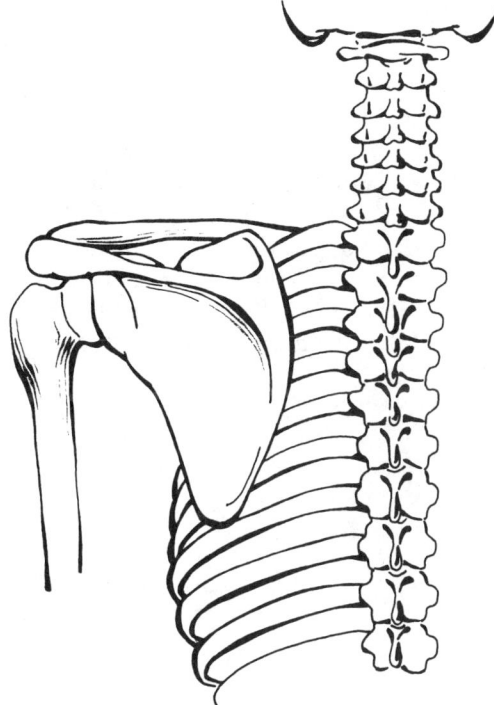

Figure 6-7

30. Teres major
    O:
    I: Inferior to lesser tuberosity of humerus, posterior to latissimus dorsi
    N: Lower subscapular n. (C-5, C-6, C-7)
    R:
    A: Extension, adduction, medial rotation of the humerus at the shoulder

31. Levator scapulae
    O: Transverse processes of atlas, axis, and 3–4 cervical vertebrae
    I:
    N: Branch of dorsal scapular n. (C-3, C-4)
    R: Slightly oblique from superior and medial origin to inferior and lateral insertion
    A: Scapular elevation

32. Rhomboids
    O:
    I:
    N: Dorsal scapular n. (C-4, C-5)
    R:
    A: Scapular retraction (adduction) with downward rotation

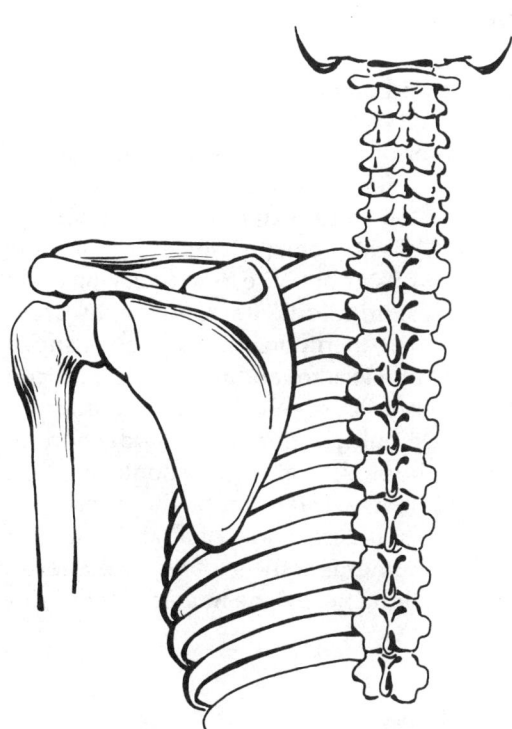

Figure 6-7

33. Latissimus dorsi

   O:
   I:
   N: Thoracodorsal n. (C-6, C-7, C-8)
   R: Fibers run inferior to superior from medial O to lateral I; Posterior to axis for flexion and extension; Wraps medially around the axis for rotation; Medial (or inferior) to axis for abduction and adduction
   A: Extension, medial rotation, adduction of the humerus at the shoulder

Figure 6-8

34. Deltoid

   O:
   I: Deltoid tuberosity of humerus
   N:
   R: Anterior fibers—slightly oblique, superior to inferior, and anterior to the axis for flexion and extension; Posterior fibers—slightly oblique, superior to inferior, and posterior to the axis for flexion and extension; Middle fibers—straight from superior to inferior, and lateral (or superior) to the axis for abduction and adduction
   A: Anterior fibers—flexion of the humerus at the shoulder; horizontal adduction of the humerus at the shoulder; Posterior fibers—extension of the humerus at the shoulder; horizontal abduction of the humerus at the shoulder; Middle fibers—abduction of the humerus at the shoulder

Figure 6-6

35. Trapezius
    O: Upper fibers—from the external occipital protuberance; medial third of the nuchal line; the ligamentum nuchae; and the posterior spinous process of the seventh cervical vertebra; Middle fibers—from the posterior spinous processes of the first through fifth thoracic vertebrae; Lower fibers—from the posterior spinous processes of the 6th through 12th thoracic vertebrae
    I: Upper fibers—to the lateral third of the clavicle and the acromion; Middle fibers—to the acromion and spine of the scapula; Lower fibers—to the vertebral end of the spine of the scapula
    N:
    R:
    A:

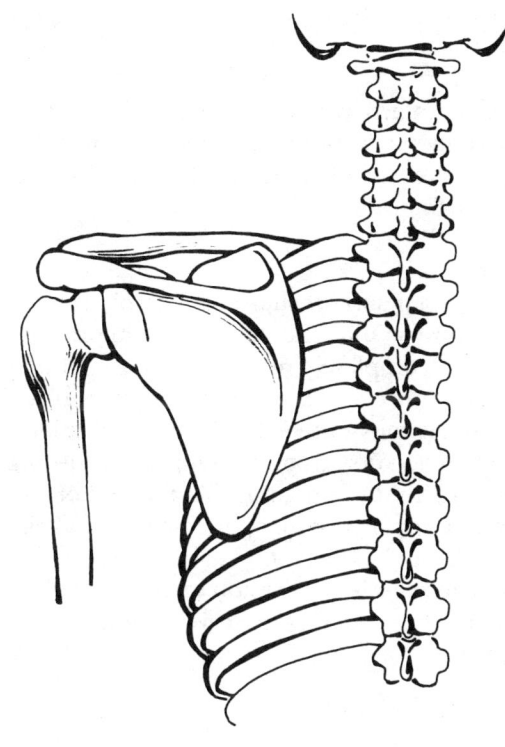

Figure 6-7

36. For the arm to accurately move in space, it must work from a stable base; in this case a stable scapula. List the muscles that stabilize the scapula on the thorax.

37. Make a list of the muscles whose lines of pull could each produce an inferior glide of the head of the humerus on the surface of the glenoid fossa. Which of these muscles actively participate with the humeral elevators during elevation of the hand above the head?

38. Which of the scapular stabilizers can perform upward rotation of the scapula?

39. What muscles can produce motion at both the shoulder and the elbow with the arm in an open kinematic chain?

40. Give the most likely antagonist for each of the following muscles:
    a. Posterior deltoid _____
    b. Serratus anterior _____
    c. Rhomboids _____
    d. Teres major _____
    e. Pectoralis minor _____

APPLICATIONS

*41. Using an articulated skeleton, examine the relationship of the greater tuberosity and the acromion during abduction without rotation of the humerus at the shoulder. What occurs with this relationship if the humerus is medially rotated during abduction? Laterally rotated?

*42. Place your subject supine on the plinth with her shoulder at the edge of the plinth. Stand on the side of the plinth near that shoulder and support the upper extremity by holding the subject's hand. Try to get your subject completely relaxed so you can move the extremity passively with no participation from the subject's musculature. Be sure to have the extremity high enough to clear the humerus from the plinth surface. Now, *passively* move the extremity into complete abduction. Be sure to move slowly and continue to obtain complete relaxation from the subject. At the beginning of the movement, you should see the anterior surface of the brachium uppermost. At the end of the range of motion you should see the medial surface of the brachium uppermost. (Uppermost means facing upward toward the ceiling.)

   Describe the motion of the humerus at the glenohumeral joint that you observed. Considering that there was no muscle contraction on the part of the subject and that you did not try to create any motion other than abduction, explain why this motion occurred. Hint: examine the configuration of the fibers of the articular capsule.

*43. Have your subject perform active extension of the humerus at the shoulder in a fashion that will allow the triceps to assist with the movement with the greatest active tension possible through the largest range of motion possible. What principle was being demonstrated?

*44. Your partner has lost function of cranial nerve XI. Muscle test the muscles directly affected, and then the movements secondarily affected.

*45. Either you or your partner perform the reverse actions of the following muscles:
   a. Latissimus dorsi
   b. Lower trapezius
   c. Pectoralis major, lower fibers

   Of what clinical significance is the ability to perform these reverse actions?

*46. Examine the scapulohumeral rhythm of your partner and decide at what point in the active range of abduction of the humerus at the shoulder the scapula first begins upward rotation. Record the goniometric value of humeral elevation at that point. Have your partner repeat this process with you. Compare the two values. How similar or different were the values? How do they compare to standard values you have found in texts for the point at which the scapula begins to move?

*47. Actively fix (hold still with your muscles) the glenohumeral joint so that no motion occurs there. Maintain the fixation and move your hand away from your body. What movements did you use to accomplish the activity? How do your observations apply to accurate manual muscle testing and goniometry of the shoulder?

*48. Position the upper extremity to place the long head of the triceps on maximum stretch.

*49. Repeat the procedure to stretch the long head of the biceps.

*50. Position the upper extremity in order to palpate the greater tuberosity of the humerus. What tendon is exposed and accessible to treatment in this position?

51. What joint is primarily affected by the costoclavicular ligament? What are the effects on that joint of a torn costoclavicular ligament?

52. Tightness in the anterior portion of the capsule of the glenohumeral joint limits lateral rotation of the humerus at the shoulder. What additional motion of the glenohumeral joint can be limited as a result of the limited lateral rotation? Why?

53. Fracture of the greater tuberosity of the humerus will directly affect the actions of what muscle? With these muscles effectively weakened, what shoulder motions will be affected and what functional activities limited?

54. Examine the anatomy of the glenohumeral joint and decide what structures would be most disrupted by an anterior-inferior dislocation of the glenohumeral joint. What are two muscles that reinforce the anterior portion of the joint? Which would you think is the stronger reinforcer of the joint?

55. Describe the two force couples of the shoulder girdle that assist in elevation of the upper extremity above the head. Give the muscles involved in each and the function accomplished by each force couple.

ANSWERS TO SHOULDER

1. There are seven bones comprising the shoulder complex:

   Two scapulae
   Two clavicles
   Two humeri
   One sternum

2. The first eight scapular items, the last four humeral items, and all clavicular and sternal items should be palpable. Check your text and have a faculty member confirm your information.

3. The glenoid fossa faces anteriorly, laterally, and superiorly in the resting shoulder girdle.

4. The humeral head is disproportionately large in relation to the glenoid fossa; the fossa is shallow. Both conditions create an unstable joint needing considerable stabilization from ligaments and muscles.

5. The sternoclavicular joint is a plane synovial joint with three degrees of freedom of movement. The movements are determined by the movement of the distal end of the clavicle and are:

   Elevation and depression
   Protraction and retraction
   Rotation

6. Check your text and have a faculty member confirm your information.

7. The SC joint disc is attached superiorly to the clavicle and inferiorly to the sternum and provides some congruity to the highly incongruous SC joint. It is interposed between the medial end of the clavicle and the sternum and allows for some contact between the superior half of the medial end of the clavicle and the sternum.

8. a. The interclavicular ligament limits depression of the clavicle.
   b. The costoclavicular ligament limits protraction, retraction, and also elevation of the clavicle.
   c. The anterior and posterior sternoclavicular ligaments reinforce the joint capsule and limit the anterior/posterior movement of the medial end of the clavicle that is associated with retraction and protraction. This movement of the medial end of the clavicle is due to the fact that the axis of rotation for protraction and retraction is through the costoclavicular ligament.

*9. a. Elevation of the clavicle accompanies scapular elevation.
   b. Depression of the clavicle accompanies scapular depression.
   c. Protraction of the clavicle accompanies scapular abduction.
   d. Retraction of the clavicle accompanies scapular adduction.
   e. Rotation of the clavicle occurs after the clavicle has completed its elevation and accompanies upward rotation of the scapula.

10. The acromioclavicular joint is a plane synovial joint with three degrees of freedom. The scapular movements include rotation in the frontal plane, winging in the horizontal plane, and tipping in the sagittal plane.

11. Check your text and, if necessary, have a faculty member confirm your information.

12. a. The coracoclavicular ligament helps maintain the integrity of the acromioclavicular joint by holding the clavicle to the coracoid process. The trapezoid portion pulls the clavicle into forward rotation as a result of scapular upward rotation that occurs past 90° of humeral elevation.
    b. The acromioclavicular ligament maintains apposition of the joint surfaces and helps prevent posterior dislocation of the clavicle on the acromion.
    c. The coracoacromial ligament closes the coracoacromial arch and prevents superior dislocation of the humeral head.

13. The glenohumeral joint is a ball and socket joint with three degrees of freedom of movement.

14. Check your text and have a faculty member confirm your information.

15. In all cases where you have manually prevented scapular movement, the humeral excursion will be less than normally expected. Full motion of the humerus requires simultaneous scapular motion.

16. Abduction of the humerus at the shoulder produces superior rolling and inferior gliding of the head of the humerus.

17. The inferiorly directed force of the rotator cuff muscles counteracts the superior rolling of the humeral head.

18. The subacromial/subdeltoid bursa is a synovial sac with potential space that extends from below the acromion to the lateral aspect of the humerus. It is superficial to the tendon of the supraspinatus and deep to the deltoid muscle. It assists in providing smooth sliding of the greater tuberosity under the acromion during humeral elevation.

19. The capsule of the glenohumeral joint attaches medially around the glenoid fossa proximal to the labrum, extends to the root of the coracoid process enclosing the proximal attachment of the biceps long head, attaches laterally at the anatomical neck of the humerus, extending a sleeve along the bicipital groove surrounding the biceps long-head tendon in the groove. The capsule is large and loose providing great range of motion and the inferior portion lies in folds when the humerus is at rest in upright posture. The inferior portion is the weakest portion of the fibrous capsule.

20. The motions of the scapula include elevation, depression, abduction (protraction), adduction (retraction), upward rotation, downward rotation, anterior tipping (rounding), posterior tipping (opposite of rounding), and winging (medial border of the scapula comes away from the chest wall).

21. Since the description is in your own words, it is impossible to give the *correct* answer here. However, you should include the aspects of humeral elevation with scapular upward rotation and humeral lowering with scapular downward rotation as well as the ratio of humeral movement to scapular movement. Also discuss the effect the scapular movement has on the length-tension relationship of the deltoid and its effect on joint congruity in the glenohumeral joint.

22. The sternoclavicular joint is the only bony attachment of the shoulder girdle to the trunk.

23. Pectoralis major, all items given in text.

24. Pectoralis minor
    O: Anterior and superior margins of the third, fourth, and fifth ribs
    I: Coracoid process of the scapula
    N: Medial pectoral n. (C-6, C-7, C-8, T-1)
    R: Fibers run upward and obliquely from medial to lateral
    A: Downward scapular rotation and anterior tipping of the scapula

25. Serratus anterior
    O: Outer superior border of 1st 8–9 ribs
    I: Ventral surface of medial border of scapula
    N: Long thoracic n. (C-5, C-6, C-7, C-8)
    R: Line of force runs from anterior on the thorax to posterior on the medial border of the scapula
    A: Scapular abduction and some upward rotation of scapula

26. Coracobrachialis
    O: Coracoid process of the scapula
    I: Middle third of the medial surface of the shaft of the humerus
    N: Musculocutaneous n. (C-6, C-7)
    R: Slightly oblique from O to I and anterior to axis for shoulder flexion and extension
    A: Flexion of the humerus at the shoulder and slight adduction

27. Supraspinatus
    O: Supraspinous fossa of the scapula
    I: Highest point of greater tubercle of humerus
    N: Suprascapular n. (C-4, C-5, C-6)
    R: Straight (horizontal) from O to I and superior and lateral to axis for abduction and adduction
    A: Abduction of the humerus at the shoulder; compression of the humeral head onto the glenoid fossa

28. Teres minor
    O: Axillary border of scapula
    I: Lowest point of greater tubercle of humerus
    N: Axillary n. (C-5, C-6)
    R: Obliquely upward from O to I; wraps around longitudinal axis posteriolaterally
    A: Lateral rotation of the humerus at the shoulder

29. Infraspinatus
    O: Infraspinous fossa
    I: Middle point of greater tubercle of humerus
    N: Suprascapular n. (C-4, C-5, C-6)
    R: Upward, oblique from O to I and wraps around laterally to the longitudinal axis
    A: Lateral rotation of the humerus at the shoulder

30. Teres major
    O: Inferior angle of scapula
    I: Inferior to lesser tuberosity of humerus; posterior to latissimus dorsi
    N: Lower subscapular n. (C-5, C-6, C-7)
    R: Oblique, superiorly from O to I and wraps medially to the longitudinal axis; medial (or inferior) to the axis for adduction and abduction; posterior to the axis for flexion and extension
    A: Extension, adduction, medial rotation of the humerus at the shoulder

31. Levator scapulae
    O: Transverse processes of atlas, axis, and 3–4 cervical vertebrae
    I: Vertebral border of scapula, superior to root of spine
    N: Branch of dorsal scapular n. (C-3, C-4)
    R: Slightly oblique from superior and medial origin to inferior and lateral insertion
    A: Scapular elevation and downward rotation

32. Rhomboids
    O: Spinous processes C-7 to T-5
    I: Vertebral border of scapula from spine to inferior angle
    N: Dorsal scapular n. (C-4, C-5)
    R: Oblique from superior to inferior from O to I and posterior and medial to the axis for adduction and abduction of the scapula
    A: Scapular retraction (adduction) with downward rotation

33. Latissimus dorsi
    O: Spines of lower 6 thoracic, lumbar, and sacral vertebrae; posterior aspect of iliac crest; three or four lower ribs; and perhaps the inferior angle of the scapula
    I: Intertubercular groove of humerus
    N: Thoracodorsal n. (C-6, C-7, C-8)
    R: Fibers run inferior to superior from medial O to lateral I; posterior to axis for flexion and extension; wrap medially around the axis for rotation; medial (or inferior) to the axis for abduction and adduction
    A: Extension, medial rotation, adduction of the humerus at the shoulder

34. Deltoid
    O: Anterior border, superior surface of lateral third of clavicle (anterior fibers), lateral margin and superior surface of the acromion (middle fibers); inferior lip of the posterior border of the spine of the scapula (posterior fibers)
    I: Deltoid tubercle of humerus
    N: Axillary n. (C-5, C-6)
    R: Anterior fibers—slightly oblique, superior to inferior and anterior to the axis for flexion and extension; Posterior fibers—slightly oblique, superior to inferior and posterior to the axis for flexion and extension; Middle fibers—straight from superior to inferior and lateral to the axis for abduction and adduction
    A: Anterior fibers—flexion of the humerus at the shoulder; horizontal adduction of the humerus at the shoulder; Posterior fibers—extension of the humerus at the shoulder; horizontal abduction of the humerus at the shoulder; Middle fibers—abduction of the humerus at the shoulder

35. Trapezius
    O: Upper fibers—external occipital protuberance; medial third of the nuchal line; the ligamentum nuchae; and the posterior spinous process of the seventh cervical vertebra; Middle fibers—posterior spinous processes of the first through fifth thoracic vertebrae; Lower fibers—posterior spinous processes of the 6th through 12th thoracic vertebrae
    I: Upper fibers—lateral third of the clavicle and the acromion; Middle fibers—acromion and spine of the scapula; Lower fibers—vertebral end of the spine of the scapula
    N: Spinal accessory n. (cranial n. XI)
    R: Upper fibers run obliquely and laterally from superior to inferior, superior to the axis for elevation; Middle fibers run horizontally from O to I, medial to the axis for adduction and abduction; Lower fibers run obliquely and laterally from inferior O to superior I, inferior to the axis for depression
    A: Upper fibers—scapular elevation; upward rotation; Middle fibers—scapular retraction (adduction); Lower fibers—scapular depression; adduction; and upward rotation

36. The primary muscles that stabilize the scapula on the thorax are those that have attachments to each, that is, trapezius (all portions), levator sapulae, rhomboids, serratus anterior, pectoralis minor.

37. The muscles that could produce an inferior glide of the humeral head on the glenoid fossa would have a line of pull that runs from inferior to superior and from either the scapula or thorax to the humerus, that is, latissimus dorsi, teres major, teres minor, infraspinatus, subscapularis, and pectoralis major (sternal fibers). The ones that participate with the humeral elevators are the teres minor, infraspinatus, and subscapularis.

38. The scapular stabilizers that also produce some upward rotation of the scapula are the upper trapezius, lower trapezius, and the serratus anterior.

39. The only two joint muscles at the shoulder and elbow are the biceps and the triceps (long head).

40. a. Antagonists to the posterior deltoid: anterior deltoid opposes extension of the humerus at the shoulder; pectoralis major opposes horizontal abduction
    b. Antagonist to the serratus anterior: rhomboids oppose scapular abduction and upward rotation
    c. Antagonist to the rhomboids: serratus anterior opposes scapular adduction and downward rotation
    d. Antagonist to the teres major: teres minor opposes medial rotation of the humerus at the shoulder; middle deltoid opposes adduction of the humerus at the shoulder; anterior deltoid opposes extension of the humerus at the shoulder
    e. Antagonist to the pectoralis minor: lower trapezius opposes anterior tipping of the scapula

*41. This activity is designed to provide a visual reference for one aspect of the biomechanics of abduction of the humerus at the shoulder. The greater tuberosity abuts the acromion during pure abduction of the humerus at the shoulder. This contact occurs earlier in the range of motion if the humerus is medially rotated, and is avoided if it is laterally rotated during the abduction movement.

*42. This activity is designed to demonstrate the role of the glenohumeral joint capsule in providing the needed lateral rotation during abduction of the humerus at the shoulder. The learners will be able to more clearly understand the result if they consult an anatomy text showing the alignment of the capsule fibers. This activity also provides kinesthetic practice to the learners who are attempting to feel the difference between partial and complete relaxation on the part of the subject.

*43. This activity reinforces the principle of two joint muscles maintaining strength of contraction through a wide range of movement. This is accomplished by preventing active insufficiency through compensatory lengthening at one joint while shortening at another joint. The participants should see the functional movement of combined shoulder extension with elbow flexion. These combined motions provide lengthening of the triceps long head over the elbow with shortening at the shoulder. This is the combined movement used in lifting a weight from the floor. The reciprocal relationship between the motions over two joints of a two-joint muscle is also demonstrated in the hamstrings and in the rectus femoris as discussed in the hip chapter (Chap. 3). Note that the biceps brachii also maintains a favorable length-tension relationship through combined shoulder extension and elbow flexion.

*44. The primary muscles to be tested are the trapezius and the sternocleidomastoid. Secondary muscles are related to the trapezius since it is a scapular stabilizer for humeral elevation. In this case, any muscle primarily responsible for humeral elevation would be tested.

*45. This activity reinforces the principle of reverse actions. In this case, the distal part is the humerus and scapula and the proximal part is the trunk. The learner stabilizes the humerus and scapula and elevates the trunk. A sitting push-up will accomplish all the reverse actions at once. One clinical significance of understanding this reverse action is understanding that these are some of the prime muscles used in crutch walking. There are many other clinically significant understandings available including the neurological levels needed to perform a sitting push-up, and so on.

*46. This activity allows for practice of shoulder goniometry, for palpation of joint and scapular motion, and for the appreciation of the variation in normal. Large discrepancies may be seen during this activity, and goniometric reliability and validity can also be discussed, as well as the value of accurate palpation and observation.

*47. This activity demonstrates the usual joint motion substitution pattern for tightness in the glenohumeral joint or weakness in a glenohumeral joint elevator muscle. The result will reinforce the value of stabilization when muscle testing the elevators of the humerus at the shoulder as well as when doing goniometry of the glenohumeral joint. In both of these activities (muscle testing and goniometry), joint motion rather than movement of the shoulder complex is the intent of the evaluation.

*48. This activity reinforces the principle of flexibility testing or stretching of a two-joint muscle, and demonstrates the position of all joints necessary to demonstrate passive insufficiency in a two-joint muscle.

*49. See item 48.

*50. To expose the greater tuberosity for easy palpation, the humerus must be extended and medially rotated at the shoulder. The rotator cuff tendon is most accessible in this position.

51. A torn costoclavicular ligament will change the axis for protraction and retraction and for elevation and depression at the sternoclavicular joint. It will also allow translatory force to be transmitted directly from the scapula to the SC joint. The first consequence will be movement at the SC joint (medial end) in the same direction as movement at the distal (acromial) end, rather than the clavicle moving in one direction on the sternum and in a different direction at the distal end. The second consequence will be greater wear and tear on the joint than there would be if the ligament were intact.

52. Abduction of the humerus will also be limited since lateral rotation is necessary for the greater tuberosity to clear the acromion.

53. The rotator cuff muscles will be affected, thus affecting lateral rotation, medial rotation, and abduction or elevation of the humerus. The rotations are obvious; the effect on abduction or elevation is because the rota-

tor cuff must be effective in order to produce a force couple with the deltoid to produce strong rotary motion of the lever, in this case elevation of the humerus. If the counter force of the rotator cuff is not effective, the deltoid will provide more translatory than rotary force.

54. The most likely structures damaged in an anterior-inferior dislocation of the shoulder would be the anterior capsule, the subscapularis muscle, and the biceps long-head tendon. Other structures frequently damaged are the anterior glenoid labrum and frequently the bony rim of the fossa. The two muscles have just been mentioned. The subscapularis has much greater mass than the biceps tendon, so we would expect that it would have a larger role in stabilizing the joint.

55. The two force couples of the shoulder complex are the scapular upward rotation couple and the humeral elevation couple. The scapular force couple is composed of the upper and lower trapezius and the serratus anterior with the center of rotation being within the scapula, but at different points during the full excursion of range of motion. When all are working in concert, upward rotation occurs. The humeral force couple consists of the deltoid pulling up and the rotator cuff pulling down with the center of rotation between the greater tuberosity and the deltoid tubercle. Such a center of rotation will produce significant downward stabilization of the head on the glenoid fossa, thus preventing the greater tuberosity from impinging on the acromion. Rotation about this center will also produce elevation of the humerus.

CHAPTER 7

Elbow and Forearm

OSTEOLOGY OF THE ELBOW AND FOREARM

*1. Identify the following structures on a laboratory partner:

Medial and lateral epicondyle of humerus
Medial and lateral supracondylar line
Olecranon process
Olecranon fossa
Ulnar border
Radial head
Ulnar nerve at elbow
Muscle bellies:
    Pronator teres
    Flexor carpi radialis

Palmaris longus
Flexor carpi ulnaris
Triceps (three heads)
Biceps brachii
Brachialis
Brachioradialis
Extensor carpi radialis longus and brevis
Extensor carpi ulnaris
Tendons of the biceps, brachialis, and triceps
Brachial artery

*2. Label the bony landmarks or prominences indicated on the following diagrams. Put a star by those that you can palpate. Make sure you can find the starred ones on your laboratory partner.

Figures 7-1 through 7-3

132

ARTHROLOGY OF THE ELBOW AND FOREARM

3. On Figures 7–4, 7–5, and 7–6, draw in the annular ligament, radial collateral ligament, ulnar collateral ligament, and the interosseous membrane.

Figures 7–4 and 7–5　　　　　　　**Figure 7–6**

4. What is the function of the interosseous membrane? Why are the fibers of the interosseous membrane aligned as they are?

5. What is the function of the annular ligament?

6. Complete the following outline:
   Humeroulnar joint
   Type of joint

   Type of motion that occurs at joint

   Amount of motion available at joint (give the range of motion normally available and degrees of freedom)

7. Complete the following outline:
   Humeroradial joint
   Type of joint

   Type of motion that occurs at joint

8. Using the convex-concave rule, describe the motions of flexion and extension of the forearm at the humeroulnar and humeroradial joints.

*9. On a laboratory partner compare the end-feels of flexion and extension of the elbow. The two should feel different. What normally limits these two motions? How would you explain the difference in the end-feels?

10. Complete the following outline:
    Proximal radioulnar joint
    Type of joint

    Type of motion that occurs at joint

11. Complete the following outline:
    Distal radioulnar joint
    Type of joint

    Type of motion that occurs at joint

12. The radioulnar joints are involved in what motions? What is the normal range for the motions?

*13. Using either loose bones or articulated models, mimic the motions of supination and pronation. Compare and describe the relative positions of the radius and ulna at the end-points of supination and pronation.

MYOLOGY OF THE ELBOW AND FOREARM

Use the following muscle sheets to aid in learning the origins, insertions, and innervations of the forearm muscles. For each of the muscles named, draw in the muscle on the sketch and complete the indicated information in the outline.

The following abbreviations apply throughout the muscle sheets:

O: Origin of muscle
I: Insertion of muscle
N: Innervation (both spinal level and peripheral nerve)
R: Relationship of muscle to axis of motion
A: Action of muscle

14. Biceps brachii
    O: Short head—coracoid process of scapula; Long head—supraglenoid tubercle of scapula
    I: Posterior aspect of radial tuberosity
    N: Musculocutaneous n. (C-5, C-6)
    R: Fibers run straight from superior O to inferior I; anterior to axis for shoulder flexion and extension (long head); anterior to axis for elbow flexion and extension; superior to and wraps around axis for supination and pronation
    A:

Figure 7–7

15. Supinator
    O: Lateral epicondyle of humerus; ulna, distal to radial notch; annular ligament and radial collateral ligament of elbow
    I: Dorsal and lateral surfaces of body of radius, distal to radial head
    N:
    R: Fibers run obliquely from superior O to inferior I; posterior to axis for pronation and supination
    A: Supination of the forearm

16. Triceps brachii
    O: Long head—
       Lateral head—
       Medial head—
    I: Posterior surface of proximal olecranon
    N: Radial n. (C-7, C-8)
    R: Fibers run obliquely, depending on head; shoulder (long head only)—posterior to axis for flexion and extension; medial to axis for abduction and adduction; elbow—posterior to axis for flexion and extension
    A: Long head—
       Lateral head—
       Medial head—

17. Brachialis
    O: Distal half of anterior surface of humerus
    I:
    N: Musculocutaneous n. (C-5, C-6)
    R:
    A: Flexion of the ulna on the humerus

18. Brachioradialis
    O:
    I: Lateral side of radial styloid
    N:
    R: Anterior to axis for flexion and extension; anterior or posterior to axis for pronation and supination, depending upon starting position of forearm
    A:

19. Pronator teres
    O: Medial epicondyle of humerus; common flexor tendon; and coronoid process
    I:
    N: Median n. (C-6, C-7)
    R:
    A:

Figure 7-8

Figure 7-7

20. Pronator quadratus
    O:
    I:
    N:
    R: Anterior to axis for pronation and supination
    A: Pronation of the forearm

Figure 7-7

APPLICATIONS

21. What are the functional implications of an adhesion between the head of the radius and the annular ligament?

*22. A patient presents with weakness of elbow flexion. Without consulting a muscle-testing textbook, demonstrate how you would differentiate between weakness in the biceps, brachialis, and brachioradialis by appropriately positioning the patient and the upper extremity to emphasize one muscle over the others.

*23. Position the subject's upper extremity to stretch the brachialis muscle without interference from a possibly tight biceps muscle. How did you confirm that your position was appropriate?

*24. Position the subject's upper extremity to put the long head of triceps on maximal stretch. How did you determine that the long head was actually on maximal stretch?

*25. Place the subject's upper extremity so that:
   a. The biceps is at a position in which it produces its weakest contraction

   b. The triceps is at a position in which it produces its weakest contraction

   c. What principle are you applying in these two activities?

*26. If the radius and ulna were fused, what joints could a person use to turn the palm of the hand up enough to accept a coin without dropping it? Demonstrate your answer. What is the importance of this observation to accurate goniometric evaluation of forearm supination and pronation?

*27. Place your subject in a position so that contraction of the biceps and anterior deltoid will extend the elbow.

28. How does the distal humerus act as a pulley for the triceps?

29. Diagram (using an end view or cross section of the radius) the mechanism by which the biceps brachii causes supination of the forearm.

*30. Demonstrate and describe the movement of the glenohumeral and humeroulnar joints that will allow the biceps to flex the elbow with strength through the largest possible range. What principle is being demonstrated in this activity?

31. Forearm supination and pronation may be limited by tightness or adhesions in which ligament(s)? Be sure to consider all relevant joints. Explain your answer.

32. Extension of the forearm at the elbow may be limited by tightness or adhesions in which ligament(s)? Be sure to consider all relevant joints. Explain your answer.

33. What muscle(s) could serve as a neutralizer for the biceps when you flex the forearm at the elbow with the forearm in pronation?

34. Assume that you would treat pain at the epicondyles of the elbow by resting the muscles attached to the epicondyle. How would your treatment of pain at the lateral epicondyle differ from treatment of pain at the medial epicondyle?

ANSWERS TO ELBOW

*1. Use your texts to identify the landmarks. Then have a faculty member confirm your palpations.

2. Check your text to confirm your information.

3. Check your text to confirm your information.

4. The purpose of the interosseous membrane is:
   a. To transfer force from the radius to the ulna, and through the ulna to the humerus
   b. To provide stability for the radioulnar joints. The alignment of fibers from proximal on the radius to distal on the ulna allows for the efficient transfer of force from the radius to the ulna. Fibers oriented in other directions provide stability of the superior and inferior radioulnar joints.

5. To maintain the head of the radius in close contact with the ulna and to stabilize the head of the radius during supination and pronation.

6. The humeroulnar joint is part of a compound synovial joint with the humeroradial joint that allows approximately 135° to 145° of active flexion and 0° of extension. This motion occurs through the gliding of the ulna around the trochlea of the humerus. There is 1° of freedom available.

   Humeroulnar joint

   Type of joint—compound synovial joint, hinge joint
   Type of motion that occurs at joint—flexion and extension by the humerus rolling within the olecranon or the olecranon rolling around the humerus
   Amount of motion available at joint (give the range of motion normally available and degrees of freedom)—135° to 145° of flexion and 0° of extension; one degree of freedom

7. **Humeroradial joint**

   Type of joint—part of a compound synovial joint with the humeroulnar joint.
   Type of motion that occurs at joint—elbow flexion and extension through the gliding of the radial head around the capitulum of the humerus. Pivoting of the radial head on the capitulum is also required for pronation and supination to occur.

8. During flexion in an open kinematic chain the concave surfaces of the radius and ulna glide anteriorly around the convex capitulum and trochlea of the humerus. During extension the surfaces glide posteriorly.

*9. Elbow extension should have a hard end-feel because the olecranon process contacts the olecranon fossa at the end of the range. The end-feel for flexion is soft or springy because the forearm flexor musculature contacts the elbow flexor musculature at the end of the range of flexion.

10. **Proximal radioulnar joint**

    Type of joint—synovial pivot joint
    Type of motion that occurs at joint—the radial head is contained within the annular ligament as it pivots on the capitulum of the humerus and the radial notch of the ulna; the resultant motion is pronation and supination of the forearm.

11. **Distal radioulnar joint**

    Type of joint—synovial pivot joint
    Type of motion that occurs at joint—the distal radius glides around the distal aspect of the ulna, allowing pronation and supination

12. Pronation and supination. Approximately 80° to 90° of each are present, though pronation is often slightly less than supination.

*13. Confirm your motions with a faculty member. Note that the proximal end of the radius rotates, but remains in the same position relative to the capitulum and proximal ulna, while the distal aspect of the radius rotates around the distal ulna, moving from the lateral aspect of the ulna in supination to the medial aspect in pronation.

14. Biceps brachii
    O: Short head—coracoid process of scapula; Long head—supraglenoid tubercle of scapula
    I: Posterior aspect of radial tuberosity
    N: Musculocutaneous n. (C-5, C-6)
    R: Fibers run straight from superior O to inferior I; anterior to axis for shoulder flexion and extension (long head); anterior to axis for elbow flexion and extension; superior to and wraps around axis for supination and pronation
    A: Elbow flexion; forearm supination

15. Supinator
    O: Lateral epicondyle of humerus; ulna, distal to radial notch; annular ligament and radial collateral ligament of elbow
    I: Dorsal and lateral surfaces of body of radius, distal to radial head
    N: Radial n. (C-6)
    R: Fibers run obliquely from superior O to inferior I; posterior to axis for pronation and supination
    A: Supination of the forearm

16. Triceps brachii
    O: Long head—infraglenoid tubercle of scapula; Lateral head—posterior humerus, proximal to groove for radial n.; Medial head—posterior surface humerus, distal aspect
    I: Posterior surface of proximal olecranon
    N: Radial n. (C-7, C-8)
    R: Fibers run obliquely, depending on head; shoulder (long head only)—posterior to axis for flexion and extension; medial to axis for abduction and adduction; elbow—posterior to axis for flexion and extension
    A: Long head—shoulder and elbow extension and shoulder adduction; Lateral and medial heads—elbow extension

17. Brachialis
    O: Distal half of anterior surface of humerus
    I: Coronoid process of ulna and ulnar tuberosity
    N: Musculocutaneous n. (C-5, C-6)
    R: Anterior to axis for flexion and extension
    A: Flexion of the elbow

18. Brachioradialis
    O: Lateral supracondylar ridge of humerus
    I: Lateral side of radial styloid
    N: Radial n. (C-5, C-6)
    R: Anterior to axis for flexion and extension; anterior or posterior to axis for pronation and supination, depending upon starting position of forearm
    A: Elbow flexion; pronation from fully supinated position to neutral; supination from fully pronated position to neutral

19. Pronator teres
    O: Medial epicondyle of humerus; common flexor tendon; coronoid process of ulna
    I: Lateral aspect of middle of radial shaft
    N: Median n. (C-6, C-7)
    R: Anterior to axis for pronation and supination; anterior to axis for elbow flexion and extension
    A: Forearm pronation; elbow flexion (assists)

20. Pronator quadratus
    O: Anterior surface of distal ulna
    I: Anterior surface of distal radius
    N: Median n. (C-8, T-1)
    R: Anterior to axis for pronation and supination
    A: Pronation of the forearm

21. If the head of the radius is not free to rotate within the annular ligament, full pronation and supination cannot occur. Where in the range of pronation and supination the limitation would occur would depend on the position of the radius when the adhesion developed.

*22. Since the biceps brachii does both supination and elbow flexion, use of this muscle can be detected by the combined motion. Brachioradialis can cause some forearm supination if the forearm is pronated and can cause some pronation if the forearm is supinated. Because of its insertion on the ulna, the brachialis does no other action with elbow flexion. By using these characteristics, the examiner can determine which muscle is working by combining forearm position and palpation during elbow flexion.

With the forearm supinated strongly, the biceps is the strongest flexor of the forearm. Its tendon can be palpated during elbow flexion in the cubital fossa.

When the forearm is pronated and the elbow is flexed, the brachialis can be palpated on either side of the biceps brachii tendon. Since supination is being voluntarily inhibited, the brain will "choose" not to have the biceps brachii participate as much in elbow flexion.

When the forearm is in neutral between pronation and supination and the elbow is flexed, the brachioradialis can easily be palpated along the radial aspect of the elbow and proximal forearm.

A knowledge of the anatomy of the muscles of elbow flexion combined with palpation of those muscles can be used to determine which muscles are working most strongly to cause elbow flexion.

*23. Since the brachialis only crosses one joint and the biceps crosses two joints, placing the biceps so that it is slack over one joint would allow the brachialis to be stretched without interference from the tight biceps. Since the brachialis only crosses the elbow joint, it must be stretched over that joint. Therefore, the biceps would need to be put in a slack position over the shoulder joint. The position of choice for this activity would be shoulder flexion and elbow extension.

*24. The proximal attachment of the long head of the triceps is the infraglenoid tubercle of the scapula. The insertion is the olecranon process of the ulna. To maximally stretch this muscle, these two points need to be separated as much as possible. This is best done with maximum shoulder flexion combined with maximum elbow flexion.

*25. a. The weakest position of the biceps would be a combination of *either* extreme shoulder flexion, extreme elbow flexion, and extreme supination *or* extreme shoulder extension, extreme elbow extension, and extreme pronation. In these positions, contraction of the biceps will produce a relatively weak contraction.
   b. The weakest positions for the triceps would be similar—extreme shoulder flexion with extreme elbow flexion or extreme shoulder extension with extreme elbow extension. Supination and pronation would not affect the strength of the triceps. In either of the positions described, elbow extension and, to some extent, shoulder extension would be weakened.
   c. The principle being applied is active insufficiency of the muscle that is being asked to contract. The positions in which a muscle is weakest are extreme lengthening and extreme shortening. This is an application of the length-tension relationship.

*26. The shoulder and the carpal joints. By abducting and adducting the shoulder a person can alter the position of the palm. The many carpal joints also allow some limited pronation and supination.

For accurate goniometry, therefore, the shoulder must be controlled and the measurement should not include motion that occurs in the carpal joints. Both of these conditions can be met by aligning one arm of the goniometer with the humerus and the other with a line formed by the distal radius and ulna (across either the anterior or posterior surface of the distal forearm, proximal to the wrist).

*27. The biceps brachii can flex the humerus at the shoulder as can the anterior deltoid. If the hand is stabilized while the elbow is flexed and the shoulder extended (as in sitting with the palm on the seat surface and elbow slightly flexed), contraction of the biceps and anterior deltoid will cause shoulder flexion. With the hand stabilized, flexion of the humerus at the shoulder will cause extension of the elbow. Other muscles would also be active in the normal individual, such as the triceps and the pectoralis major. But if the triceps was not able to function, active elbow extension could still be accomplished in the manner described above, though it would not be particularly strong.

28. The distal humerus is angled anteriorly in comparison to the shaft of the humerus. This angulation causes the axis of motion of elbow flexion to be displaced anteriorly, which effectively increases the moment arm for the line of pull of the triceps.

29. The head of the radius is held next to the ulna by the annular ligament. During pronation and supination the head of the radius rotates within this ligament. The biceps branchii inserts on the tuberosity of the radius. In pronation the tuberosity is oriented more posteriorly which wraps the tendon of the biceps around the radius (Figs. 7–9 and 7–10). Upon contraction, the biceps causes the radius to "unwind" or supinate (Figs. 7–9 and 7–10). It can be diagramed as follows.

Figures 7–9 and 7–10

*30. By starting the motion with the humerus flexed moderately at the shoulder and the elbow extended, and then simultaneously extending the humerus at the shoulder and flexing the forearm at the elbow, the length-tension relationship of the biceps brachii is maintained in a stronger range. This will allow increased strength through the typically weaker end ranges of elbow motion. These motions will keep the biceps relatively stretched over one joint as it shortens over the other joint. This is an application of the length-tension relationship.

31. Since the interosseous membrane, the anterior radioulnar ligament, and the oblique cord all limit supination, abnormal limitation in any of them can cause decreased supination. The posterior radioulnar ligament limits pronation, so abnormal limitation of this ligament can cause decreased pronation. Excessive tightness of the annular ligament can also limit pronation and supination. It should be noted, however, that pronation is normally more limited by bony approximation than by ligamentous tightness.

32. Tightness of the anterior joint capsule, the anterior portions of the ulnar and radial collateral ligaments, and any of the muscles crossing the anterior surface of the elbow joint have the potential to decrease elbow extension. Tightness in these anterior structures would not allow the posterior motion of the radius and ulna over the distal portion of the humerus that is required for extension.

33. The two muscles that pronate the forearm are the pronator teres and the pronator quadratus. Either or both of these muscles could neutralize the supination component of the biceps brachii during elbow flexion.

34. You must first determine what muscles attach to each area. The medial epicondyle generally serves as an attachment for the wrist and finger flexors. The lateral epicondyle serves as an attachment for the wrist and finger extensors.

Pain at the lateral epicondyle might be treated by resting the wrist and finger extensors. Remember that the wrist extensors are a strong synergist for the finger flexors. In fact, more extensor activity is probably generated by this synergy than primary use of the extensors. Therefore, finger and wrist flexion may also need to be limited. Pain at the medial epicondyle, on the other hand, would require rest of the wrist and finger flexors.

CHAPTER 8

The Wrist and Hand

OSTEOLOGY AND ARTHROLOGY OF THE WRIST AND HAND

*1. Identify the following landmarks or structures on a laboratory partner.

Radial styloid
Ulnar styloid
Pisiform
Hook of hamate
Scaphoid
Triquetrum
Capitate
Sesamoid bones of thumb
Base, shaft, and head of each metacarpal
Base, shaft, and head of each phalanx
Joint line of MCP (metacarpophalangeal)
    and PIP (proximal interphalangeal) joints

Flexor retinaculum
Tendons:
    Flexor carpi ulnaris
    Flexor carpi radialis
    Extensor carpi radialis longus and brevis
    Extensor carpi ulnaris
    Interossei (palmar and dorsal)
    Flexor digitorum superficialis and profundus
    Extensor digitorum
    Extensor indicis
    Extensor digiti minimi

2. Complete the following outline in relation to the joints of the wrist and hand:

   Wrist joint (radiocarpal joint)

   Bones involved

   Type of joint

Name(s) of motion(s) at joint

Amount of motion available at joint

Midcarpal joints
Bones involved

Type of joint

Name(s) of motion(s) at joint

Amount of motion available at joint

Carpometacarpal joint of thumb
Bones involved

Type of joint

Name(s) of motion(s) at joint

Carpometacarpal joints of fingers
Bones involved

Type of joint

Name(s) of motion(s) at joint

Metacarpophalangeal joint
Bones involved

Type of joint

Name(s) of motion(s) at joint

Amount of motion available at joint

Interphalangeal joints
Bones involved

Type of joint

Name(s) of motion(s) at joint

Amount of motion available at joint

NEUROLOGY OF THE WRIST AND HAND

3. Describe the peripheral nerve sensory distribution to the hand. Why are we asking you about the sensory distribution in the hand when we have not mentioned sensory considerations in any other area?

4. Describe the peripheral nerve motor distribution to the intrinsic muscles of the hand. What is the relationship of the innervation of the intrinsics and the extrinsics?

MYOLOGY OF THE WRIST AND HAND

Use the following muscle sheets to aid in learning the origins, insertions, and innervations of muscles of the wrist. For each of the muscles named, draw in the muscle on the sketch and complete the indicated information on the outlines.

O: Origin of muscle
I: Insertion of muscle
N: Innervation (both spinal level and peripheral nerve)
R: Relationship of muscle to the axis of motion
A: Action of muscle

Muscles of the Wrist

5. Extensor carpi radialis longus
   O:
   I: Dorsal surface, base of index metacarpal
   N:
   R: Posterior to axis for flexion and extension of wrist; radial to axis for abduction and adduction of wrist
   A: Wrist extension; wrist radial deviation (limited)

6. Extensor carpi radialis brevis
   O: Lateral epicondyle of humerus
   I:
   N: Radial n. (C-6, C-7)
   R:
   A: Wrist extension

7. Extensor carpi ulnaris
   O: Lateral epicondyle of humerus
   I: Ulnar side of base of fifth metacarpal
   N:
   R:
   A:

Figure 8–1 Figure 8–1

8. Flexor carpi ulnaris
   O:
   I:
   N: Ulnar n. (C-8, T-1)
   R: Palmar to axis for flexion and extension of wrist; ulnar to axis for abduction and adduction; anterior to axis for flexion and extension of elbow
   A:

9. Flexor carpi radialis
   O: Medial epicondyle of humerus
   I:
   N:
   R:
   A: Wrist flexion; wrist radial deviation; elbow flexion

Extrinsic Muscles of the hand

10. Extensor digitorum
    O:
    I:
    N:
    R: Dorsal to axes for flexion and extension of MCPs, IPs, and wrist; neutral to axes for abduction and adduction of wrist, MCPs, and IPs
    A: Wrist extension; MCP extension; IP extension

11. Extensor indicis
    O: Dorsal surface of ulna distal to thumb extensor
    I:
    N: Radial n. (C-6, C-7, C-8)
    R: Posterior to axes for flexion and extension of MCP and IP; neutral to axis for abduction and adduction of MCP; posterior to axis for flexion and extension of wrist
    A:

12. Extensor digiti minimi
    O: Lateral epicondyle of humerus
    I: Extensor mechanism of fifth digit
    N:
    R: Dorsal to axes for flexion and extension of MCP and IP; neutral to axis for abduction and adduction of MCP
    A:

Figure 8-2

Figure 8-1   Figure 8-1

13. Extensor pollicis brevis
    O: Distal third of dorsal surface of radius
    I:
    N: Radial n. (C-6, C-7)
    R: Posterior to axis for MCP flexion and extension; dorsal to axis for wrist flexion and extension; radial to axis for wrist abduction and adduction
    A:

14. Extensor pollicis longus
    O:
    I: Base of distal phalanx of thumb, dorsal surface
    N: Radial n. (C-6, C-7, C-8)
    R: Dorsal to axes for flexion and extension of wrist, MCP, IP; radial to axis for abduction and adduction of wrist; neutral to axis for abduction and adduction of thumb MCP
    A:

15. Abductor pollicis longus
    O: Dorsal surface of middle of both ulna and radius
    I: Radial side of base of first metacarpal
    N:
    R:
    A: Abduction of MC (metacarpal carpal) joint of thumb; radial deviation of wrist; flexion of wrist

16. Flexor digitorum superficialis
    O:
    I:
    N:
    R: Neutral to axes for abduction and adduction of wrist and MCP; palmar to axes for flexion and extension of wrist, MCPs, and PIPs
    A: PIP flexion of digits 2–5; MCP flexion of digits 2–5; wrist flexion

17. Flexor digitorum profundus
    O:
    I:
    N: Digits 2, 3—median n. (C-8, T-1); digits 4, 5—ulnar n. (C-8, T-1)
    R: Palmar to axes for wrist, MCP, PIP, DIP (distal interphalangeal) flexion and extension; neutral to axis for abduction and adduction of wrist and MCP
    A:

Figure 8-1   Figure 8-1

Figure 8-2   Figure 8-2

18. Flexor pollicis longus
    O:
    I:
    N: Median n. (C-8, T-1)
    R:
    A: Flexion of thumb MCP; flexion of thumb IP; wrist flexion; radial deviation of wrist (minimal)

Figure 8-2

Intrinsic Muscles of the Hand

19. Opponens pollicis
    O:
    I: Radial side of length of first metacarpal
    N:
    R: Medial to axis for flexion and extension of MC joint thumb; palmar to axis for abduction and adduction of MC joint; ulnar to axis for rotation of MC joint
    A:

20. Opponens digiti minimi
    O:
    I: Ulnar side of fifth metacarpal
    N: Ulnar n. (C-8, T-1)
    R: radial to axis for opposition of fifth metacarpal joint
    A:

21. Abductor digiti minimi
    O: Pisiform; tendon of flexor carpi ulnaris
    I:
    N: Ulnar n. (C-8)
    R:
    A: MCP ulnar deviation; MCP flexion

Figure 8-3

22. Dorsal interossei

   O:
   I:
   N: Ulnar n. (C-8, T-1)
   R: Palmar to axis for flexion and extension of MCP; radial to axis for abduction and adduction of index and long fingers; ulnar to axis for abduction and adduction of long and ring fingers
   A:

23. Adductor pollicis

   O:
   I: Base of proximal phalanx of thumb
   N: Ulnar n. (C-8, T-1)
   R:
   A:

24. Abductor pollicis brevis

   O: Scaphoid; trapezium; transverse carpal ligament
   I:
   N: Median n. (C-6, C-7)
   R: Radial to axis for abduction and adduction of MCP; radial to axis for abduction and adduction of MC joint
   A:

25. Flexor pollicis brevis

   O:
   I: Base of proximal phalanx, palmar surface
   N: Radial portion—median n. (C-6, C-7); Ulnar portion—ulnar n. (C-8, T-1)
   R: Palmar to axes for flexion of MCP and IP of thumb
   A: Thumb MCP and IP flexion

26. Palmar interossei

   O:
   I:
   N: Ulnar n. (C-8, T-1)
   R: Palmar to axis for MCP flexion and extension; index—ulnar to axis for abduction and adduction of MCP; ring and little—radial to axis for abduction and adduction of MCP; dorsal to axes for flexion and extension of IP joints
   A:

27. Lumbricals

   O:
   I: Radial aspect of extensor mechanism of each finger at the level of the MCP joint
   N: First and second lumbricals—median n. (C-6, C-7); Third and fourth lumbricals—ulnar n. (C-8)
   R:
   A:

Figure 8-3

Figure 8-3

APPLICATIONS

28. What is the purpose of the sheaths surrounding the flexor tendons?

*29. Use a string to represent your flexor digitorum profundus. Tape the string to the pad of a fingertip. Pull on the string to represent a contraction of the long flexor.

   a. What happens to the string when you pull it and allow your finger to flex?

   b. What keeps this from happening with the "real" tendons in your finger?

   c. What would happen if the restraining structures in b were not intact?

*30. Review the definition of *synergy* and demonstrate two synergies that normally occur when using the hand.

31. Label the indicated items on the diagram of the extensor mechanism below.

Figure 8-4

*32. Demonstrate the "intrinsic position" (the position the fingers assume when the lumbricals and interossei are contracting simultaneously or they are shortened)?

*33. In what position would you place the fingers in order to stretch the intrinsic muscles? Do the motion on yourself and feel for any tightness.

*34. What is the functional significance of loss of the median nerve at the wrist level (remember to consider both sensory and motor problems that might occur)? To simulate the sensory deficit, get a pair of surgical gloves. Turn one inside out. Cut the small and ring fingers off the gloves. Put both gloves on one hand. Now put your gloved hand in your pocket or pocketbook and find a quarter or some other small object that you know is there. Can you tell a quarter from a nickel without looking? Describe how you chose to identify the coins or objects? Don't forget to simulate the lack of median-innervated musculature.

*35. What is the functional significance of loss of the ulnar nerve at the wrist level (remember to consider both sensory and motor problems that might occur)? Again, use surgical gloves to simulate the loss of sensation. Alter a new set of gloves to cover the area of skin innervated by the ulnar nerve. Don't forget to simulate the lack of ulnar-innervated musculature.

36. Based on activities 34 and 35, do you think a median or an ulnar nerve lesion at the wrist level would be more debilitating in functional terms? Give your rationale.

37. What symptoms would you expect to see with edema in the carpal tunnel and why?

*38. Have a laboratory partner firmly grip two of your fingers. Now, have your partner do the same thing with her wrist in *extreme* flexion. Repeat this one more time with *extreme* wrist extension. Which was strongest, which was weakest, and why?

*39. What is a major benefit of having the extrinsic finger flexors and extensors crossing multiple joints?

*40. What would be the effect of scarring in the flexor sheath of a single finger?
   a. What is the effect of this limitation on making a fist?
   b. Give a rationale.

41. Go to your texts and review the musculotendinous anatomy of the flexor digitorum profundus and superficialis.
   a. What is a primary difference in the structure of the two muscles?
   b. With the back of your right hand on a table, immobilize your right ring finger in complete MCP, PIP, and DIP extension while you flex your index, long, and little MCPs with your left hand. Try to flex your right index, long, and little finger PIPs and DIPs in this position. What happened at the PIPs, why? What happened at the DIPs, why?
   c. Relate this finding to muscle testing to isolate the superficialis from the profundus.

ANSWERS TO WRIST AND HAND

*1. Check your text to find these items and then have a faculty member confirm your information.

2. **Wrist joint (radiocarpal joint)**
   Bones involved—radius, radioulnar disc, triquetrum, lunate, and scaphoid (navicular)
   Type of joint—synovial, condyloid
   Names of motions at joint—flexion and extension (more limited), and radial and ulnar deviation (more available)
   Amount of motion available at joint—the various components of the wrist joint are not able to be measured separately for their contributions to wrist motion. Total wrist motion is approximately 80° to 90° of flexion, 75° to 85° of extension, 15° of radial deviation, and 45° of ulnar deviation. Note that the radiocarpal joint allows more radial and ulnar deviation than flexion and extension.

   Midcarpal joint
   Bones involved—scaphoid, lunate, and triquetrum proximally; trapezium, trapezoid, capitate, and hamate distally
   Type of joint—complex of synovial plane joints
   Names of motions at joints—flexion and extension (more available), and radial and ulnar deviation (more limited)
   Amount of motion available at joints (See comments for radiocarpal joint. Note that the midcarpal joint allows more flexion and extension than radial and ulnar deviation.)

Carpometacarpal joint of thumb

Bones involved—trapezium and first (or thumb) metacarpal
Type of joint—synovial, saddle
Names of motions at joint—flexion and extension, abduction and adduction, rotation, opposition

Carpometacarpal joints of fingers

Bones involved—distal carpal row and bases of second (or index finger) through fifth (or small finger) metacarpals
Type of joint—synovial, plane
Name of motion at joint—flexion and extension

Metacarpophalangeal joint

Bones involved—metacarpal and proximal phalanx of each finger
Type of joint—synovial, condyloid
Names of motions at joint—flexion and extension, radial and ulnar deviation
Amount of motion available at joint—approximately 85° to 105° of flexion, 20° to 30° of extension, and 20° to 25° each of radial and ulnar deviation

Interphalangeal joints

Bones involved—adjacent phalanges for each finger. Note that the index, long, ring, and small fingers each have a proximal and a distal interphalangeal joint, while the thumb has only one interphalangeal joint.
Type of joint—synovial, hinge
Name of motion at joint—flexion and extension
Amount of motion available at joint—proximal interphalangeal joints (PIPs) have from 100° to 110° of flexion and typically extend to neutral without hyperextension. Distal interphalangeal joints (DIPs) typically have 80° to 90° of flexion and extend to neutral or slightly beyond.

3. The median nerve provides sensation for the thenar half of the palm and the palmar surface of the thumb, index, long, and half of the ring finger. The ulnar nerve innervates the rest of the palmar surface of the hand. The radial nerve innervates the dorsum of the hand, though there is a great deal of overlap with the median and ulnar nerves on the dorsum of the hand.

    The hand is the primary organ that interacts with the environment. Sensation is needed for protection and information gathering. Sensory information is transmitted along the sensory components of the peripheral nerves.

4. The lumbricals are innervated by the same nerve that innervates the flexor digitorum profundus muscle to which the lumbrical is attached (i.e., lumbricals 1 and 2 are innervated by the median nerve and lumbricals 3 and 4 are innervated by the ulnar nerve). All of the interossei are innervated by the ulnar nerve. The thenar muscles, with the exception of the adductor pollicis and the deep head of the flexor pollicis brevis which are innervated by the ulnar nerve, are innervated by the median nerve.

5. Extensor carpi radialis longus

    O: Distal part of lateral supracondylar ridge
    I: Dorsal surface, base of index metacarpal
    N: Radial n. (C-6, C-7)
    R: Posterior to axis for flexion and extension of wrist; radial to axis for abduction and adduction of wrist
    A: Wrist extension; wrist radial deviation (limited)

6. Extensor carpi radialis brevis

    O: Lateral epicondyle of humerus
    I: Dorsal surface, base of long metacarpal
    N: Radial n. (C-6, C-7)
    R: Posterior to axis for flexion and extension of wrist; neutral to axis for abduction and adduction of wrist
    A: Wrist extension

7. Extensor carpi ulnaris
    - O: Lateral epicondyle of humerus
    - I: Ulnar side of base of fifth metacarpal
    - N: Radial n. (C-6, C-7, C-8)
    - R: Posterior to axis for flexion and extension of wrist; ulnar to axis for abduction and adduction of wrist
    - A: Wrist extension; wrist ulnar deviation

8. Flexor carpi ulnaris
    - O: Medial epicondyle of humerus; proximal dorsal surface of ulna
    - I: Pisiform; base of fifth metacarpal
    - N: Ulnar n. (C-8, T-1)
    - R: Palmar to axis for flexion and extension of wrist; ulnar to axis for abduction and adduction of wrist; anterior to axis for flexion and extension of elbow
    - A: Wrist flexion; wrist ulnar deviation; elbow flexion

9. Flexor carpi radialis
    - O: Medial epicondyle of humerus
    - I: Base of index metacarpal, palmar surface
    - N: Median n. (C-6, C-7)
    - R: Palmar to axis for flexion and extension of wrist; radial to axis for abduction and adduction; anterior to axis for flexion and extension of elbow
    - A: Wrist flexion; wrist radial deviation; elbow flexion

Extrinsic Muscles of the Hand

10. Extensor digitorum
    - O: Lateral epicondyle of humerus
    - I: Four tendons, one to extensor mechanism of each finger
    - N: Radial n. (C-6, C-7, C-8)
    - R: Dorsal to axes for flexion and extension of MCPs, IPs, and wrist; neutral to axes axis for abduction and adduction of wrist, MCPs, and IPs
    - A: Wrist extension; MCP extension; IP extension

11. Extensor indicis
    - O: Dorsal surface of ulna distal to thumb extensor
    - I: Ulnar aspect of extensor digitorum to index extensor mechanism
    - N: Radial n. (C-6, C-7, C-8)
    - R: Posterior to axes for flexion and extension of MCP and IP; neutral to axis for abduction and adduction of MCP; posterior to axis for flexion and extension of wrist
    - A: MCP extension; IP extension; wrist extension

12. Extensor digiti minimi
    - O: Lateral epicondyle of humerus
    - I: Extensor mechanism of fifth digit
    - N: Radial n. (C-6, C-7, C-8)
    - R: Dorsal to axes for flexion and extension of MCP and IP; neutral to axis for abduction and adduction of MCP
    - A: MCP extension; IP extension; wrist extension

13. Extensor pollicis brevis
    - O: Distal third of dorsal surface of radius
    - I: Base of first phalanx of thumb, dorsal surface
    - N: Radial n. (C-6, C-7)
    - R: Posterior to axis for MCP flexion and extension; dorsal to axis for wrist flexion and extension; radial to axis for wrist abduction and adduction
    - A: Wrist extension; wrist radial deviation; MCP extension of thumb

14. Extensor pollicis longus
    O: Lateral part of middle third of body of ulna, dorsal surface
    I: Base of distal phalanx of thumb, dorsal surface
    N: Radial n. (C-6, C-7, C-8)
    R: Dorsal to axes for flexion and extension of wrist, MCP, IP; radial to axis for abduction and adduction of wrist; neutral to axis for abduction and adduction of thumb MCP
    A: Wrist extension; wrist radial deviation; thumb MCP extension

15. Abductor pollicis longus
    O: Dorsal surface of middle of both ulna and radius
    I: Radial side of base of first metacarpal
    N: Radial n. (C-6, C-7)
    R: Palmar to axes for thumb abduction and wrist flexion; radial to axis for abduction and adduction of wrist
    A: Abduction of MC joint of thumb; wrist radial deviation; wrist flexion

16. Flexor digitorum superficialis
    O: Medial epicondyle of humerus; coronoid process; palmar surface of mid-third of radius
    I: Tendons divide to insert on radial and ulnar aspects of volar surface of middle phalanges of digits 2–5
    N: Median n. (C-7, C-8, T-1)
    R: Neutral to axes for abduction and adduction of wrist and MCP; palmar to axes for flexion and extension of wrist, MCPs, and PIPs
    A: PIP flexion of digits 2–5; MCP flexion of digits 2–5; wrist flexion

17. Flexor digitorum profundus
    O: Palmar surface of base of proximal three-quarters of ulna
    I: Palmar surface of base of distal phalanges of digits 2–5
    N: Digits 2, 3—median n. (C-8, T-1); digits 4, 5—ulnar n. (C-8, T-1)
    R: Palmar to axes for wrist, MCP, PIP, DIP flexion and extension; neutral to axes for abduction and adduction of wrist and MCP
    A: Wrist flexion; MCP flexion; PIP flexion; DIP flexion

18. Flexor pollicis longus
    O: Palmar surface of middle third of radius; coronoid process of ulna
    I: Palmar surface of base of distal phalanx of thumb
    N: Median n. (C-8, T-1)
    R: Palmar to axis of flexion and extension of wrist; radial to axis of abduction and adduction of wrist; palmar to axes of flexion and extension of MCP and IP of thumb
    A: Flexion of thumb MCP; flexion of thumb IP; wrist flexion; radial deviation of wrist (minimal)

Intrinsic Muscles of the Hand

19. Opponens pollicis
    O: Trapezium; flexor retinaculum
    I: Radial side of length of first metacarpal
    N: Median n. (C-6, C-7)
    R: Medial to axis for flexion and extension of MC joint of thumb; palmar to axis for abduction and adduction of MC joint; ulnar to axis for rotation of MC joint
    A: MC oppostion (flexion, abduction, rotation)

20. Opponens digiti minimi
    O: Hook of hamate; flexor retinaculum
    I: Ulnar side of fifth metacarpal
    N: Ulnar n. (C-8, T-1)
    R: Radial to axis for oppostion of fifth MC joint
    A: Oppostion of MC joint of little finger

21. Abductor digiti minimi
    O: Pisiform; tendon of flexor carpi ulnaris
    I: Ulnar side of first phalanx of fifth finger; extensor mechanism
    N: Ulnar n. (C-8)
    R: Ulnar to axis for abduction and adduction of MCP; palmar to axis for flexion and extension of MCP
    A: MCP ulnar deviation; MCP flexion

22. Dorsal interossei
    O: Adjacent sides of metacarpals
    I: Extensor mechanism (extensor hood) and base of proximal phalanges of index, long, and ring fingers: index—radial side; long—both sides; ring—ulnar side
    N: Ulnar n. (C-8, T-1)
    R: Palmar to axis for flexion and extension of MCP; radial to axis for abduction and adduction of index and long fingers; ulnar to axis for abduction and adduction of long and ring fingers; dorsal to axes for flexion and extension of IP joints
    A: MCP flexion; MCP deviation: index—radial; long—both; ring—ulnar; IP extension

23. Adductor pollicis
    O: Capitate and bases of index and long metacarpals; shaft of long metacarpal, palmar surface
    I: Base of proximal phalanx of thumb
    N: Ulnar n. (C-8, T-1)
    R: MCP—volar to axis for flexion and extension; MC—ulnar to axis for abduction and adduction
    A: MC adduction; MCP flexion

24. Abductor pollicis brevis
    O: Scaphoid; trapezium; transverse carpal ligament
    I: Radial side of base of first phalanx of thumb
    N: Median n. (C-6, C-7)
    R: Radial to axis for abduction and adduction of MCP; radial to axis for abduction and adduction of MC joint
    A: MC and MCP abduction

25. Flexor pollicis brevis
    O: Flexor retinaculum; trapezium; ulnar border of first metacarpal
    I: Base of proximal phalanx, palmar surface
    N: Radial portion—median n. (C-6, C-7); Ulnar portion—ulnar n. (C-8, T-1)
    R: Palmar to axes for flexion of MCP and IP of thumb
    A: Thumb MCP and IP flexion

26. Palmar interossei
    O: Palmar surface of length of index, ring, and little metacarpal
    I: Side of base of proximal phalanx of corresponding finger: index—ulnar side; ring and little—radial side; extensor expansion of each digit
    N: Ulnar n. (C-8, T-1)
    R: Palmar to axis for MCP flexion and extension; index—ulnar to axis for abduction and adduction of MCP; ring and little—radial to axis for abduction and adduction of MCP; dorsal to axes for flexion and extension of IP joints
    A: MCP flexion; MCP deviation: index—ulnar; long—radial; small—radial; IP extension

27. Lumbricals
    O: Tendons of flexor digitorum profundus of each finger
    I: Radial aspect of extensor mechanism of each finger at the level of the MCP joint
    N: First and second lumbricals—Median n. (C-6, C-7); Third and fourth lumbricals—Ulnar n. (C-8)
    R: Palmar to axis for MCP flexion and extension; dorsal to axes for IP flexion and extension
    A: MCP flexion; IP extension

28. To decrease resistance of friction so that the tendons may glide easily.

*29. a. The string pulls away from your phalanges and "bows" across the finger and palm.
   b. The flexor retinaculum and the vaginal ligaments.
   c. The vaginal ligaments are designed to hold the tendons that pass under them close to the bone. If they were not there the tendons would be able to pull away from the bone (bowstringing). The shortest distance between two points is a straight line (as you saw in a above). If the flexor tendons were not held tightly to the phalanges, when the fingers were flexed in a fist the tendons would attempt to pass in a straight line from their insertion to the palm, causing the skin to "web." The grip strength would be greatly compromised since so much of the muscle's force would be used to shorten the muscle belly.

*30. One definition of synergy is muscles that work together for a common goal either by assisting each other (biceps and brachialis), by stabilizing for each other (scapular muscles for glenohumeral motion), or by neutralizing unwanted motions (rotator cuff and deltoid).

  Grip or finger flexion is usually accompanied with wrist extension (stabilizing or neutralizing). Finger extension, conversely, is usually accompanied by wrist flexion (stabilizing or neutralizing). Flexor digitorum superficialis and profundus work together to produce strong flexion of the PIP joints.

31. Here is a labeled diagram of the extensor mechanism.

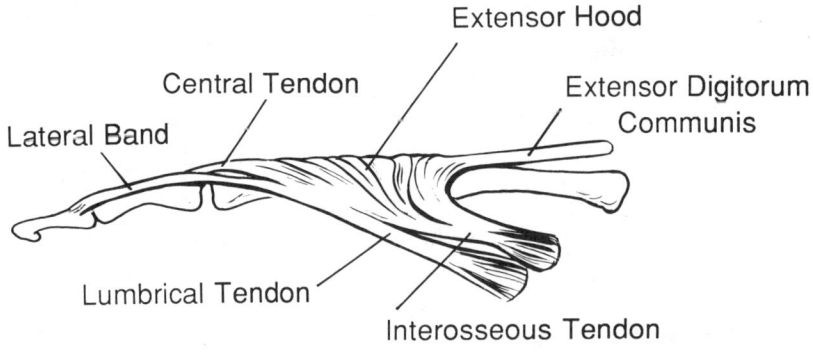

Figure 8–5

*32. MP flexion and IP extension. This is the shortened position of the intrinsic musculature.

*33. MP extension and IP flexion.

*34. Loss of the median nerve at the wrist results in a loss of sensation over the median nerve distribution of the hand and loss of muscle function of the abductor pollicis brevis, opponens pollicis, part of flexor pollicis brevis, and first two lumbricals. Functionally, this would not allow the person to position the thumb out of the plane of the palm and opposition would be almost impossible. This motor deficit severely hampers the manipulative ability of the hand.

  The sensory loss is a major handicap because we depend so heavily on sensory input in the function of the hand. The manipulative aspects of the hand are the thumb, index, and long finger pads, and all of these surfaces are innervated by the median nerve.

*35. Loss of the ulnar nerve at the wrist would result in a loss of sensation over the ulnar nerve distribution and loss of muscle function of the adductor pollicis, part of the flexor pollicis brevis, the interossei, and the two ulnar lumbricals. The weakness involved with ulnar nerve problems interferes with the ability to open or close the fingers in a broad arc. Rather than a coordinated opening that allows one to grasp a wide object, the fingers curl into the palm, pushing objects out of the palm. Curling the fingers into the palm means that all DIP and PIP flexion is completed first and it is followed by MCP flexion. In normal grasp there is coordinated and simultaneous MCP, PIP, and DIP flexion. Try to pick up a drink can by first flexing your PIPs and DIPs and then flexing your MCPs.

  The functional significance of the sensory loss is that the ulnar aspect of the hand often comes into contact with the environment (resting on surfaces). Without sensation, an individual may not know whether the environment is safe (a table top) or hostile (a stove top).

36. There is no correct answer to this. With a median nerve loss, there is sensory loss to the finger and thumb pads primarily used for interacting with the environment and inability to lift the thumb from the plane of the palm, eliminating fine prehension. With an ulnar nerve loss, there is a sensory deficit over the ulnar aspect of the hand, and the person is only able to curl and uncurl the fingers (movement in a wide arc is not possible). See item 35 for a description of curling of the fingers.

   Which injury is worse is debatable, but either one significantly affects function. Generally, however, patients seem to have more limited function with a median nerve injury than an ulnar nerve injury.

37. Edema would increase the pressure in the carpal tunnel. The structure in the tunnel most sensitive to increased pressure is the median nerve. The symptoms would be those of entrapment (interference with nerve transmission). The first symptoms are usually sensory disturbances in the median distribution of the hand. If the pressure continues, muscle weakness in the median innervated intrinsic musculature can result.

*38. Typically, the strongest grip position is the position that your partner chose without any instructions from the activity. The strongest position for finger flexion is usually mild wrist extension. The positions of extreme wrist flexion or extension will usually create weaker grip strength because of a less than optimal length-tension relationship.

*39. By crossing many joints, the wrist and hand can have much finer control of the length-tension relationship of the extrinsic musculature. When one joint needs to be in a certain position for a specific activity, there are still several other joints that can be adjusted to maintain an optimal length-tension relationship.

   Since the extrinsic muscles of the hand are multijoint muscles, they are highly sensitive to active and passive insufficiency. In extreme wrist flexion with active finger flexion, the finger flexors are actively insufficient and the finger extensors are often passively insufficient. In extreme wrist extension with finger extension, the finger flexors are often passively insufficient and the finger extensors are actively insufficient. The strongest position for finger flexion is usually mild wrist extension and the strongest position for finger extension is mild wrist flexion.

*40. Scarring in the flexor sheath acts as a tether and limits gliding of the tendon within the sheath. Depending where the tendon and sheath are adherent, flexion, extension, or both can be limited.
   a. Making a fist would be limited.
   b. The flexor digitorum profundus muscle belly tends to pull on all fingers simultaneously. Adhesions of the profundus in one finger, therefore, could limit excursion of the other fingers, though to a lesser degree. The flexor digitorum superficialis, on the other hand, has much more independence of finger function than the profundus. Scarring of a superficialis tendon in one finger would probably not have much of an effect on the other fingers.

41. a. The profundus has one muscle belly with four interdependent tendons. The superficialis has muscle bellies that are more separated and more independent.
   b. Most people cannot flex the DIP joints in this position. The PIPs flex readily. This position effectively immobilizes the profundus tendon of the ring finger, which simulates scarring in the sheath of the ring finger. Since the profundus has one muscle belly to activate four tendons, the limitation of one tendon limits the motion in all four tendons.
   c. Using the position described in this exercise, you can effectively eliminate the contribution of the profundus muscle to flexion of any finger. This allows you to assess the strength of the superficialis. Free flexion of the fingers is the result of both profundus and superficialis function.

CHAPTER 9

Temporomandibular Joint

OSTEOLOGY OF THE TEMPOROMANDIBULAR JOINT

*1. Palpate the following structures on a laboratory partner and label them on Figure 9–1.

Mandible
    Condyle (from lateral aspect of face)
    Condyle (from external auditory meatus)
    Coronoid process
    Angle
    Ramus
    Body
Zygomatic arch
Hyoid bone

Figure 9–1

*2. Observe your partner for facial symmetry. Are eyes and ears level? Are the nose and mouth in the center of the face? Is the mandible centered? Observe at least three people. Did you find symmetry or asymmetry more often?

ARTHROLOGY OF THE TEMPOROMANDIBULAR JOINT

*3. The following diagrams demonstrate the two components of joint motion during mouth opening. First the condyle rotates in the mandibular fossa (Figures 9–2a and b) and then it glides downward and forward over the articular eminence (Figures 9–2b and c). Using a skull and a mandible, demonstrate both of these motions.

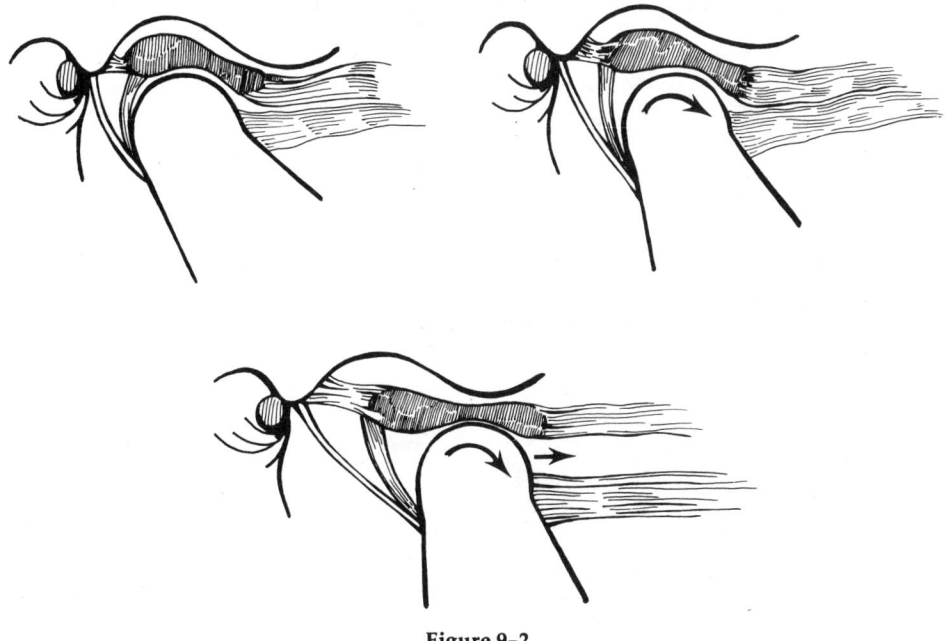

Figure 9–2

*4. On a laboratory partner, palpate the temporomandibular joint on mouth opening and mouth closing. Two methods of palpation are (1) place your fingers lightly just anterior to the ear lobes and request that the person open and close the mouth gently, and (2) place your little finger inside the external auditory meatus and palpate the anterior aspect of the canal as the mouth opens and closes. Can you feel when rotation and translation occur in the range of motion? Did the joints move symmetrically? Did you feel any popping or clicking?

5. If you were to observe someone with a normal TMJ opening and closing his mouth, would you expect to see any lateral deviation?

6. The mandible has two articulations, one at each condyle. What are the implications of this arrangement on independent joint motion.

7. A disc covers the condyle like a sock. Consult texts and describe the attachments of the disc to the condyle and to other structures.

8. Describe how the disc moves during normal mouth opening and closing.

*9. On at least three laboratory partners, observe normal jaw movement and determine how you might measure it. The movements you want to observe and measure are mouth opening and closing, lateral deviation to each side, protrusion (jutting the jaw forward), and retrusion (sliding the jaw backward). Describe your measurement technique. Measure the laboratory partners using the methods you develop. What ranges of motion did you observe?

*10. On at least three laboratory partners observe for lateral deviation of the mandible during mouth opening and closing. Choose a landmark (the spaces between the front teeth are often convenient) and ask the subject to open and close his mouth slowly. Do the two points you are observing keep the same relation throughout the motion? If they do not, what is the deviation?

MYOLOGY OF THE TEMPOROMANDIBULAR JOINT

*11. Palpate the following muscles on a laboratory partner:

Masseter   Suprahyoid muscles
Temporalis   Scalenes (anterior, middle)
Infrahyoid muscles Sternocleidomastoid

Use the following muscle sheets to aid in learning the origins, insertions, and innervations of the muscles of the TMJ. For each of the muscles described, find its placement on a skull.

O: Origin of muscle
I: Insertion of muscle
N: Innervation (both spinal level and peripheral nerve)
R: Relationship of muscle to axis of motion
A: Action of muscle

12. Masseter

O: Zygomatic arch
I: Coronoid process, ramus, and angle of mandible
N: Trigeminal n.—cranial n. V
R: Anterior to axis for elevation and depression
A: Elevates mandible

Figure 9–3

13. Temporalis
    O: Temporal fossa and fascia
    I: Coronoid process and anterior border of ramus of mandible
    N: Trigeminal n.—cranial n. V
    R: Anterior to axis for elevation and depression
    A: Elevates and retracts mandible

Figure 9–4

14. Medial pterygoid
    O: Medial surface of lateral pterygoid plate
    I: Medial surface of ramus and angle of mandible
    N: Trigeminal n.—cranial n. V
    R: Translatory motion, axis irrelevant; muscle in line with motion
    A: Unilateral action: protrusion and lateral deviation to the opposite side; Bilateral action: elevation of mandible

15. Lateral pterygoid
    O: Sphenoid and lateral surface of lateral pterygoid plate
    I: Front of condyle of mandible; anterior portion of the disc, and capsule of joint
    N: Trigeminal n.—cranial nerve V
    R: Translatory motion, axis irrelevant; muscle in line with motion
    A: Unilateral action: protrusion and deviation to opposite side; bilateral action: lower portion active during mandibular depression, superior portion active during mandibular elevation

Figure 9–5

16. Digastric
    - O: Mastoid
    - I: Through pully attached to hyoid to posterior aspect of center of mandible
    - N: Facial n.—cranial n. VII
    - R: Posterior to axis for elevation and depression
    - A: Depresses the mandible or elevates the hyoid

See also:

All neck musculature
Sternocleidomastoid
Scalenes (anterior, posterior, middle)

Figure 9-6

17. Describe the forces that control the motion of the disc during normal mouth opening and closing. Refer to your answer to item 8 in completing this item.

APPLICATIONS

18. If the disc dislocates posteriorly, what motion of the condyle would be limited? If the disk dislocates anteriorly, what motion of the condyle would be limited? Explain why these limitations occur.

*19. What would be the effect of an injury or obstruction that allowed only the rotation component of joint motion during mouth opening to occur in the left temporomandibular joint (TMJ). Assume that the right TMJ has normal motion. What would you see on mouth opening and closing? Recreate these problems with a skull and mandible.

*20. Describe the jaw motion on opening and closing that you would expect to see in the following two people:
Ophelia has a tight joint capsule of the left TMJ that limits translation.
Cadwallader has an anteriorly dislocated left disc that reduces on mouth opening and dislocates on mouth closing.

*21. Sit with erect posture (normal primary and secondary curves). In that position, gently tap your teeth together and feel where they touch. Now put your chin on your chest and tap your teeth together. Look at the ceiling and tap your teeth together. Finally, tap your teeth together while you are in a forward head posture. The last two positions are quite similar in both the occiput-atlas relationship and their effect on how the teeth meet (occlusion). Most people find that their teeth touch in different places in the different head positions.
   a. Based on this exercise, describe the association between head position and occlusion. Record the relationship of your teeth in each of the positions (e.g., lower teeth forward of regular bite).

   b. Why might this occur? (You will need to know the myology of the TMJ to answer this.)

   c. Management of TMJ dysfunction includes physical therapy and dental techniques. The dental techniques are often intended to change the patient's occlusion (bite). How should PT (physical therapy) and dental intervention be sequenced?

ANSWERS TO TEMPOROMANDIBULAR

*1. Check your texts to find these structures and then have a faculty member confirm your palpations.

*2. Use this exercise to practice facial-observation skills. You will most likely find many examples of asymmetry. Mild asymmetry is the norm and is of no consequence functionally. You may find some examples of marked asymmetry which are still of no functional consequence. You may also find some deviations which could be functionally significant. Have a faculty member confirm your observations.

*3. Make sure you demonstrate, see, and feel the two distinct motions involved in mouth opening.

*4. Use this exercise to practice your palpation skills. You may find several examples of asymmetrical movement and popping or clicking.

5. No lateral deviation is usually seen during mouth opening and closing in an individual with a "normal" TMJ. Many instances of lateral deviation do occur that are totally asymptomatic and should not be treated.

6. When one articulation is affected by anything, the other articulation will also be affected. Since the connection between the two articulations is rigid (the mandible), any stress or force on one joint will be transmitted in some manner to the other joint.

7. Medially and laterally the disc is attached firmly to the poles of the condyle of the mandible; there are no medial or lateral attachments of the disc to the capsule. The anterior portion of the disc is attached to the capsule and the superior portion of the lateral pterygoid muscle. The posterior aspect of the disc is attached to the bilaminar retrodiscal pad. This pad is composed of two bands. One band is attached to the tympanic plate through elastic fibers; the other band is attached to the neck of the condyle and is not elastic.

Figure 9-7   Figure 9-8

8. During normal mouth opening, the disc rotates posteriorly on the condyle during the rotation phase of the motion and then glides forward with the condyle during the translation phase of the motion. On closure, the process is reversed. First the disc and condyle glide posteriorly, and then the disc rotates anteriorly over the condyle to return to the initial closed-mouth position.

*9. A person can typically place the width of three of his own PIP joints between the upper and lower teeth. An opening of two PIP joints is functional. This measurement is too gross for specific evaluation of TMJ function, but it can be an effective "home assessment" for the patient.

    The most common method of measuring joint motion is by using a ruler to measure the motion (in millimeters) in each direction. Generally accepted ranges of motion are 40 to 50 mm of opening and 8 mm of lateral deviation to each side.

*10. Use this exercise to practice observational skills. Have a faculty member confirm your observations.

*11. Have a faculty member confirm your palpations.

12 to 16. The completed outlines were provided in the myology section of the workbook.

17. During the rotation phase of normal mouth opening, the disc is restrained by the posterior attachments of the disc, which causes a posterior rotation of the disc in relation to the condyle. During the translation phase of mouth opening, the disc moves forward with the condyle by virtue of its firm attachments to the condylar poles. The inferior lamina of the retrodiscal pad limits forward excursion of the disc. See Figures 9–7 and 9–8 in the answer to item 7 (page 170).

   During mouth closing, the disc is pulled posteriorly by the elastic fibers of the superior lamina of the retrodiscal pad. The superior portions of the lateral pterygoid muscles contract eccentrically to control the posterior motion of the disc.

18. A posteriorly dislocated disc limits mandibular elevation (mouth closing) by providing a mechanical block that does not allow the condyle to assume its normal position in the joint space.

   An anteriorly dislocated disc, on the other hand, limits mandibular depression (mouth opening) by not allowing the condyle to slide into a fully opened position. The rotation component is permitted, but the translation component is not complete.

*19. If only rotation is allowed to occur on the left as the person begins opening the mouth, normal symmetrical motion occurs until the rotation phase is complete. As the person tries to continue opening the mouth, translation will occur on the right but will be unavailable on the left, causing the mandible to deviate to the left. This occurs because translation is continuing on the right, but no motion is occurring on the left. Make sure you recreate this motion using a skull and mandible. See Figure 9–9.

Figure 9–9

*20. The tight capsule limiting translation would create the same clinical picture as described in item 19. On mouth opening, Ophelia would have a C curve to the left.

   Cadwallader's motion, however, would be uneven. At first, on opening, Cadwallader's motion would be symmetrical. At the end of rotation the mandible would deviate to the left as the disc limited translation on the left and translation occurred on the right. At the point when the disc would reduce (or relocate), the mandible would "jump" back to the midline as the translation on the left would be completed. On closure the movement would also be uneven. As closure started, the movement would be even until the disc dislocated. At that point the mandible would deviate to the left until the normal translation on the right was completed. As the translation on the right is completed the mandible would be returning to the midline. The rotation phase of closing would probably be symmetrical. Individual variations from this general description will be determined by tightness or looseness of the joint capsule and ligaments.

In summary, a tight joint capsule will create a C curve to the same side, while a dislocated disk will create a complex curve. Make sure you recreate these motions using a skull and mandible in order to gain a fuller understanding of the mechanism of the joint.

*21. a. During extension of the head on the neck, the mandible tends to retract (move posteriorly in relation to the maxilla). During flexion, the mandible tends to protrude (move anteriorly in relation to the maxilla).
   b. This could be caused by tight musculature or soft-tissue impingement. For instance, extension of the head on the neck would tend to stretch the digastric, which would tend to retract the mandible. On the other hand, in extreme flexion of the head and neck, the soft tissues of the neck tend to push the mandible into a more protruded position.
   c. A forward-head posture is often present in a person with TMJ dysfunction. Physical therapy procedures are designed to affect posture, muscle length, strength, and coordination. These procedures will often affect (decrease) the forward head position of the patient. As this exercise has demonstrated, head position can affect occlusion (how the teeth come in contact with each other). Therefore, the physical therapist should see the patient early. If the PT is not involved in the case until after the dentist has completed work with the patient's occlusion, a great deal of dental work may need to be redone as the patient's occlusion changes through the PT treatments.

CHAPTER 10

Posture

APPLICATIONS

Static posture results from the alignment of the body's segments so that the composite center of mass becomes vertically aligned over the base of support.

*1. On your laboratory partner, place colored stick-on markers on surface landmarks that will allow you to analyze her standing posture from the lateral and posterior views.

2. Describe the ideal standing posture of the body from a lateral and a posterior view.

3. You will be using a plumb line to examine the vertical relationship of the surface landmarks marked in item 1. To place the plumb line in a consistent manner among subjects, you need a consistent point of reference with which to align the plumb line. For this activity, you will be viewing posture from the lateral and the posterior aspects, therefore you will need a lateral and a posterior landmark for use as your point of reference for each view.

   Determine a logical point of reference for the lateral view and for the posterior view for your postural analysis.

*4. Compare the posture of five of your classmates with the ideal you described in item 2. Be sure to use the lateral and posterior views on each subject. In addition to the reference-point landmark for the posterior view you chose in item 1, include the following bilateral assessments in your comparison:

Shoulder height
Orientation of scapula
Space between elbow and waist
Height of iliac crests
Gluteal folds
Popliteal creases
Medial malleoli

5. What lines define the lumbosacral angle and what is the normal angle formed by those lines?

*6. Demonstrate an increased lumbosacral angle in the standing position.

7. Describe the posture of the hips and lumbar spine in the position you assumed in item 6. Use the Rule of Three.

*8. Demonstrate a decreased lumbosacral angle in the standing position.

9. Describe the posture of the hips and lumbar spine in the position you assumed in item 8. Use the Rule of Three.

*10. Examine normal posture from a lateral view using a plumb line and the landmarks you identified in item 1. From the normal standing position, place a 3-in elevation under the subject's heels. What changes occur in the relationship of each landmark to the plumb line? Now place the elevation under the balls of the feet. What changes occur in the relationship of each landmark to the plumb line?

11. On Figure 10–1, assume the vertical line represents the line of gravity.

Figure 10-1

a. What motion is the force of gravity attempting to produce at each lower extremity joint?

b. What muscles at the hip and knee are responsible for counteracting this effect of gravity?

*12. Assume the position drawn in Figure 10–1 and maintain it until you feel contraction in the hip and knee muscles responsible for maintaining the posture. Are they the same muscles you listed in item 11?

13. On Figure 10–2, assume that the vertical line represents the line of gravity. What is the effect of gravity at the hip and at the knee?

Figure 10–2

a. Contrast the effect of gravity on the hip and the knee in Figures 10–1 and 10–2. Include a discussion of the relative magnitude of the effect as seen in each figure.

b. Which posture requires greater energy to maintain?

14. Given that the primary and secondary curves of the spine act as shock absorbers for vertical compression of the spine, what effect will decreasing the lumbosacral angle have on the shock absorption capacity of the lumbar spine?

*15. Have your partner sit in a chair and be sure she assumes a relaxed position. Describe her lumbosacral angle in this sitting position.

*16. Do what you need to do in order to bring her lumbosacral angle in sitting back to a normal angle. Once you have corrected the lumbosacral angle, provide her with sufficient support so that she can relax and maintain the angle while sitting. State what you did to affect the angle.

*17. While standing, assume a forward-head posture. Have a classmate verify the posture. What criteria did you use to determine what the posture would look like?

*18. In the sitting position have your partner assume a pronounced forward-head posture. Now, have her raise her sternum. To do this she will need to imagine that a vertical string is pulling her sternum up toward the ceiling. You should see her ribs rise as her sternum elevates. What effect did raising the sternum have on the forward-head posture? Would this work in a standing position?

*19. Have your partner stand with as close to ideal posture as possible. Observe her spinal curves from the lateral view. Now, have her stand with a forward-head posture and note the spinal curves. Describe what you saw.

20. Explain how the forward-head posture places the bilateral sternocleidomastoid muscles in a shortened position.

21. On Figure 10–3, place a force vector representing the effect of gravity on the head. What deviations from ideal posture do you note in the illustration?

Figure 10-3

*22. The weight of the human head is between 10 and 15 lb. Hold a 10-lb weight in your hand and rest your elbow on the table with your forearm vertical. Extend your wrist with the weight resting in your open palm. Hold this position for 2 minutes. At the end of the 2 minutes, describe the sensation you feel in your wrist.

23. Explain the result of item 22 in terms of the torque produced by gravity on the weight in your hand and the effort of the muscles responsible for counteracting that torque.

24. Relate items 21 and 23.

25. Name the curves in the scolioses illustrated in Figures 10–4 and 10–5.

Figure 10-4

Figure 10-5

*26. Place a dot over the spinous processes of all the palpable vertebrae on your partner. From a posterior view, evaluate the spine for deviations from vertical alignment. Have your partner bend forward. Does the alignment change in any way? Evaluate for scoliosis or rib humps. What view would you use to evaluate for kyphosis or flattening of the primary or secondary curves?

*27. Have your partner stand with a 1-in elevation under the right foot, keeping both knees fully extended. From a posterior view, evaluate how this alters her posture.

28. What direction will the thoracic vertebrae rotate with right lateral bending of the thoracic spine? Which direction will the spinous processes move in conjunction with that vertebral rotation? If the right lateral bend is fixed, as in structural scoliosis, on which side will the posterior rib hump be noticed? Explain.

*29. In a public place, observe the posture of an individual who has a protruding abdomen, for example, a pregnant woman. Describe how this affects the individual's standing posture. Determine how this would affect the muscles responsible for maintaining the erect posture.

*30. Have your partner lie supine on a table and have her try to make one leg look longer than the other. What motion did she perform to accomplish this miraculous feat? Devise a measurement scheme to determine whether the leg is actually longer or some other explanation of this phenomenon exists.

*31. Measure segmental versus total leg length. What landmarks did you use to measure each segment? Discuss the reason for measuring both total length and segmental length, and a possible difficulty with using only one of those measurements.

ANSWERS TO POSTURE

*1. Your kinesiology text will likely show a lateral and posterior view of standing posture with a vertical line of gravity passing through the center of mass. Body landmarks typically used to examine posture will be named and located in relation to the vertical line. Some standard surface landmarks for the lateral view are ear, acromion, greater trochanter, knee, and lateral malleolus. Landmarks for the posterior view are nuchal eminence, spinous process of C-7, gluteal cleft, midpoint between the feet.

2. In the ideal posture of the human body, the line of gravity falls close to most joint axes. The body segments are in near vertical alignment, the compression forces are optimally distributed over weight-bearing surfaces. In particular, in a lateral view the line of gravity falls with the following relationships to joints and landmarks:

   Slightly anterior to axis for flexion and extension of the head on the neck and through the external auditory meatus

   Posterior to the lordotic curve of the cervical spine

   Along the lateral border of the trunk and anterior to the kyphotic curve of the thoracic spine; posterior to the lordotic curve of the lumbar spine

   Slightly posterior to the axis of flexion and extension of the hip and roughly through the greater trochanter

Slightly anterior to the axis for flexion and extension of the knee
Slightly anterior to the axis for dorsiflexion and plantar flexion of the ankle and slightly anterior to the lateral malleolus

From a posterior view: The line of gravity will ideally bisect the body into left and right halves following the spinous processes and falling from the nuchal eminence through the gluteal cleft and arriving on the floor half way between the feet.

3. The most typical landmark for consistent placement of the plumb line for a lateral assessment of posture is just anterior to the lateral malleolus. The most used landmark for consistent assessment of posture in a posterior view is the nuchal eminence. Once the plumb line has been placed over either of these landmarks, the remaining surface landmarks are examined with respect to where they fall in relation to the vertical line.

*4. This exercise allows you to appreciate the range of normal as well as assess classmates who may fall outside the range of normal. Frequently, a student is identified with a postural defect that had not been previously identified. This can be an uncomfortable situation which may need faculty input and supervision.

When examining the posterior view, the additional items listed allow for examination of symmetry between sides of the body in the frontal plane.

5. The lumbosacral angle is the angle formed by a line drawn parallel with the ground and another line drawn parallel to the superior plateau of the first sacral vertebra in the lateral view. The normal angle is about 30°.

*6. An increase in the lumbosacral angle is caused by anterior tilting of the sacrum (pelvis).

7. Flexion of the pelvis at the hip and an increase in anterior lumbar convexity (increased lumbar lordosis).

*8. A decreased lumbosacral angle is produced by a posterior pelvic tilt.

9. Extension of the pelvis at the hip and a decrease in the anterior lumbar convexity (decreased lumbar lordosis).

*10. The 3-in elevation under the heels will tend to cause the landmarks to move anteriorly. This anteriorly displaces the center of mass and thus anteriorly displaces the line of gravity in relation to the base of support. You should see the subject make an effort to move the center of mass posteriorly by increasing the lumbar lordosis and/or flexing the knees. When the elevation is placed under the toes, the reverse takes place. You may see the hips flex or some other effort to anteriorly displace the center of mass.

11. a. Hip and knee flexion; ankle dorsiflexion
    b. The hip extensors (gluteus maximus and hamstrings) are most responsible for resisting the force of gravity at the hip; the quadriceps are responsible for resisting the force of gravity at the knee.

*12. Sense the tension in the muscles listed in item 11.

13. a. Item 11 illustrates gravity producing a flexor moment at the hip and knee while Figure 10–2 demonstrates the line of gravity falling slightly behind the axis for flexion and extension of the hip and slightly in front of the axis for flexion and extension of the knee. This alignment produces an extensor moment at each joint. The line of gravity falls further away from the joint in item 11 (Figure 10–1) than in Figure 10–2, making the moment arm of the gravity force greater in item 11. With the greater moment arm and equivalent force, the torque in item 11 is greater than in item 13.
    b. The combination of less torque and the turning moment being toward the stability of each joint makes the effort to maintain the posture in Figure 10–2 much less than the posture in Figure 10–1.

14. When the lumbosacral angle is decreased, more force from the weight of the upper body mass is transmitted directly to the vertebral bodies and intervertebral disks causing increased compression. Normally, the force is dissipated by the lumbar curve.

*15. The typical lumbosacral angle in sitting is decreased since the sacrum is more posteriorly tilted.

*16. You will most likely provide some support for the posterior lumbar spine so the normal lordotic curve reappears. The position will allow your partner to sit erect but relaxed.

*17. The simplest criterion is relative placement of the head on the neck, which is effectively assessed by the position of the zygomatic arch (cheekbone) over the manubrium. The commonly used alignment of the auditory canal over the acromion can be misleading if the individual has both a forward head and rounded shoulders. The rounding of the shoulders may place the acromion under the external auditory meatus, even with forward head posture.

*18. Raising the sternum typically reduces the forward head. Yes, it will also apply in the standing position.

*19. Jutting the head forward increases the kyphotic posture of the thoracic spine and may increase or decrease the lordotic posture of the lumbar spine. The cervical spine shows flexion in the lower segments and extension in the upper segments.

20. The sternocleidomastoid (SCM) muscle crosses posterior to the axis for flexion and extension of the head on the atlas and anterior to the axis for flexion and extension of the lower cervical spine. Since the forward-jutting position extends the head on the atlas and flexes the lower cervical spine on the thorax, this combination shortens the SCM over both ends.

21. Deviations from ideal posture include kyphosis and forward head.

Figure 10-6

*22. You will most likely feel a sense of overstretching and fatigue in the muscles controlling the wrist.

23. The force of gravity falls posterior to the axis for flexion and extension producing an extension moment at the wrist. The wrist flexors attempt to counterbalance this torque, but in a mechanically disadvantageous position.

24. Fatigue and strain can occur in the posterior muscles of the neck and upper back when they are required to maintain the head upright against a flexion moment of the force of gravity, as in item 21. This is analogous to the result in the wrist in item 23.

25. The scoliosis diagrams demonstrate a left lumbar, right thoracic curve (Fig. 10–4) and a left thoracolumbar curve (Fig. 10–5).

*26. Often, if a subject shows a mild lateral curve in standing, it will disappear in forward bending, indicating that it is a functional (not fixed) curve. If the curve should remain on forward bending, then it is considered to be structural (fixed). The lateral view is necessary to see changes in the primary and secondary curves.

*27. A unilateral lift under the right foot with the right knee straight transmits the effect of the elevation directly to the lumbosacral junction. The pelvis will tip laterally, the right iliac crest will be higher than the left, and you may see a left lumbar curve in the spine. This exercise simulates the effect of the right leg being longer than the left, standing with bilateral knees extended.

28. Right lateral bend in the thoracic spine produces left rotation of the vertebrae. With left rotation of the vertebrae you observe movement of the spinous processes to the right. The ribs will follow the vertebrae, so the right ribs will move forward and the left ribs back as the vertebrae rotate to the left. If the right lateral bend is fixed as in a structural scoliosis, then there will be a posterior rib hump on the left because the curve of the left ribs has moved back and become fixed with the fixed vertebrae.

*29. A disproportionate amount of weight placed anteriorly to the normal center of mass will cause a compensatory posterior displacement of the upper trunk. This adjustment is most obvious in the lumbar spine. To maintain this posture, the lumbar spinal extensors may be overactive.

*30. This movement is accomplished by lateral tipping of the pelvis. Most of your patients, however, will not try to make one leg longer than the other. To determine whether one leg is longer than the other, or whether the pelvis is tipped, you must compare the measurements of both the bony length of the leg and the length from midline of the trunk (usually the navel).

Differences demonstrated in the measurement from the midline of the trunk may be due to lateral tipping of the pelvis, since the tipping will move the leg with the pelvis. Differences found when measuring the length of the leg itself [e.g., from the anterior superior iliac spine (ASIS) to the medial malleolus] discounts the effect of pelvic tipping and would demonstrate bone-length differences.

*31. You should be able to pick proximal and distal bony landmarks on the thigh and on the lower leg to use to measure each bone. Measuring segmentally allows you to determine which bone is short, when a short leg is noted. However, segmental measuring can increase the error in the measurement. Total leg length measured from ASIS (anterior superior iliac spine) to medial malleolus is better for eliminating errors, but determining the offending bone or segment is more difficult.

Assessing knee height with the subject supine and hips flexed to 90° (feet off the table, knees flexed) can give a visual estimate of comparative femur length, assuming no large pelvic anomaly and the pelvis is not rotated on the lumbar spine.

Assessing knee height with the subject supine and hips and knees flexed, but both feet flat on the examining table, will give a visual estimate of comparative tibial length, as the tibia are now supporting the height of the knee.

These two screening techniques can assist in determining the short segment(s) of the lower limb, if a short leg is suspected, by placing the respective rigid lever between the knee and supporting surface.

CHAPTER 11

Gait

PHASES OF GAIT

Gait and ambulation are the terms used for human locomotion. The normal gait pattern is divided into two phases.

1. Name the two phases of gait.

2. The subdivisions of each gait cycle have been described using various terms. The two most common terminology systems are the traditional (more standard) and the newer RLA (Rancho Los Amigos) system. Using the lists below, match the standard terminology of gait with the RLA terminology for gait.

Traditional	Traditional	RLA	RLA
Heel strike	Acceleration	Terminal swing	Loading response
Toe-off	Deceleration	Preswing	Midswing
Foot flat	Midstance	Initial contact	Terminal stance
Heel-off	Midswing	Initial swing	Midstance

3. On Figure 11–1, label each subdivision of the phases of gait for the *right lower extremity* using the traditional nomenclature.

Figure 11–1

184

4. Describe the relative position of the major joints of the lower extremity in each subdivision of gait. On the chart below, the descriptions for heel strike are completed as an example.

	Hip	**Knee**	**Ankle**
a. Heel strike:	Flexion	Full extension	Neutral
b. Foot flat:			
c. Midstance:			
d. Heel-off:			
e. Toe-off:			
f. Acceleration:			
g. Midswing:			
h. Deceleration:			

5. Describe the movement of the shoulder girdle and upper extremities in concert with the lower extremities.

6. Considering the right lower extremity, at which subdivisions of the gait cycle does each of the two periods of double support occur?

7. At which part of the gait cycle is the knee in maximal flexion?

DISTANCE AND TIME VARIABLES

8. How is stride length determined?

9. Contrast stride length and step length.

10. How is the velocity of gait determined?

11. Discuss the relationship between cadence and length of the period of double support.

*12. Ask a subject to stand without moving on a large piece of paper. Draw an outline of the base of support in standing. Now, have the subject mimic midstance. Draw an outline of the base of support during midstance. Finally, have the subject mimic the position during double-limb support (R-heel strike, L-heel off). Draw an outline of the base of support during double-limb support. How did you determine the size and shape of each drawing?

13. Compare the differences in widths of the standing base of support between a child and a young adult; between a young adult and an elderly adult. To what do you attribute the differences? (Note: If there is no easy reference from which to create your description, use observation of the public in an area such as a shopping plaza or theater.)

14. What is the normal degree of toe-out during gait?

    a. How does the normal degree of toe-out change with increased speed of gait?

    b. How does the degree of toe-out relate to the size of the base of support?

    c. How does the size of the base of support relate to static stability?

    d. What is the relationship of static stability to mobility?

    e. What is a possible function of the change in degree of toe-out with increased speed?

*15. For this activity you will need powder, a carpeted surface for walking, a chair, a long string, a goniometer, and a ruler. In a sitting position with your feet dangling, place powder on the plantar surface of your bare feet. Stand up with your feet a comfortable distance apart. From this position, walk through at least two full gait cycles on the carpeted surface. Come to a complete stop on the last cycle.

    a. Using a line between the medial borders of consecutive right-heel prints, measure the degree of right toe-out during ambulation versus the degree of toe-out when you came to a standing position. How can you account for the difference in degrees, if there was a difference?

    b. Measure the stride length and step width.

DETERMINANTS OF GAIT

*16. Standing behind a partner, lightly place your hands on both sides of his pelvis (iliac crests). Have your partner walk while you continue to feel the movement of the pelvis during ambulation. Make sure you do not inhibit your partner's normal gait motion. Describe the movement of the pelvis during gait.

*17. Repeat item 16, but have your partner walk with the feet close together (decreased medial and lateral base of support), then with the feet spread far apart. How does this affect the movement of the pelvis? Describe how this affects the relationship of the center of gravity and the base of support.

*18. Demonstrate how pelvic rotation in the horizontal plane over a stationary femur on the stance limb effectively lengthens the swinging limb.

19. How does the pelvic rotation described in item 18 affect the energy requirement of gait?

20. Describe how movement of the center of gravity affects the expenditure of energy during the gait cycle.

21. Explain how lack of knee flexion can increase the energy cost of gait.

22. During stance, the pelvis drops slightly toward the unsupported side. The interaction of pelvic drop with knee extension at midstance decreases the energy cost of ambulation. Explain.

23. The angle of inclination of the femoral neck on the shaft was discussed in the hip chapter (Chap. 3). What effect does this angle have on the base of support in the standing position?

24. What angle at the knee compensates for the effect of the femoral angle of inclination thus preventing the feet from crossing each other in the standing position?

25. The interaction of knee and ankle motion during gait tends to shorten the *stance* limb from heel strike to midstance and tends to relatively lengthen it from midstance to toe-off. What is the effect of this on the movement of the center of mass during stance?

26. Based on items 18 to 25, what are the six determinants of gait?

27. Why are the determinants of gait important for efficient ambulation?

MYOLOGY OF GAIT

28. During which subdivision of gait are the dorsiflexors of the ankle most active?

   a. What type of contraction are they performing?

   b. What is the function of this contraction?

29. The gastrocnemius-soleus complex is quite active from just prior to midstance to heel-off.
    a. What joint motion at the ankle is occurring from midstance to heel-off?

    b. What is the function of this contraction of the gastrocnemius-soleus group?

    c. What type of contraction is it?

30. Why is a contraction of the quadriceps necessary at heel strike?

31. Explain why the hamstrings are active during both deceleration and heel strike.

32. What is the function of the gluteus maximus in the early stance phase of gait?

33. During which subdivision of gait are the hip flexors most active? What function are they performing?

34. What is the function of the abductor muscles of the stance hip during heel strike and early stance? In what fashion do these muscles contract during heel strike and early stance?

35. In which subdivision of gait are the erector spinae muscles most active?

MOMENTUM

*36. a. Walk *very slowly* for about 20 ft. Think about how the muscles around your hips, knees, and ankles feel.
   b. Walk at a normal pace and think about how the muscles around your hips, knees, and ankles feel.
   c. Walk at normal speed. Stop suddenly on one foot. What happens to your body or balance? Think about how the muscles around your stance hip, knee, and ankle feel.
   d. What is an explanation of the difference in muscle activity you felt between a and b?

   e. Explain what happened to your body position or balance and what you felt in c.

   f. What inferrences concerning the role of momentum in normal gait can you make as a result of items a through e?

37. Item 36 demonstrates the value of momentum in maintaining forward propulsion in gait. Examine normal gait and identify which joint motions during gait are primarily caused by momentum. Identify as many sources of momentum as you can.

APPLICATIONS

*38. In groups of five, select two subjects in the group to walk so the other group members can observe normal gait. The subjects should be in laboratory clothes.
   a. Determine bony landmarks on which to apply markers to enhance the observation of joint motion in the sagittal and frontal planes. In making your choices, be sure to include markers that will allow you to view tibial and pelvic rotation in the horizontal plane and elevation and depression of the center of mass. Apply the markers.
   b. Have one subject walk at a time so all members get a chance to observe normal gait. The subject should walk normally at a moderate rate. Have the subject walk while the other members in the group record

what is occurring at each joint during each subdivision of the gait cycle. Observers will find it most effective to focus on one joint at a time and to change the focus of observation in an orderly fashion—either from the foot up or from the head down.

   c. Include in your description for b what motion is occurring at each joint from one point to the next in the gait cycle.

   d. Observe the elevation and depression of the center of mass during gait. Determine at what subdivisions of the gait cycle the center of mass is highest and lowest.

*39. Have a subject mimic severe weakness in the left gastrocnemius-soleus. The stride length of which limb will be most affected by the weakness? Why?

40. At what other point of the gait cycle, in addition to heel strike, will you be able to easily see the effect of a weak tibialis anterior?

41. What foot and ankle muscles can assist the action of a weak tibialis anterior?

42. Motion at what joints near the ankle will mask the effect of fusion of the talocrural joint?

*43. Demonstrate a gait pattern for each of the following muscle weaknesses:
   a. Bilateral gluteus maximus
   b. Unilateral gluteus medius
   c. Bilateral iliopsoas
   d. Unilateral quadriceps
   e. Unilateral pretibial group

*44. Use a low cart or board with wheels underneath (like a scooter board) to examine Newton's three laws of motion. In the following examples, the scooter board becomes a barometer of applied force and the relative reactions to applied forces. The following activities are designed to demonstrate the three laws of motion. These activities are courtesy of Dr. D. Michael McKeough, Associate Professor in the Department of Physical Therapy, Medical College of Georgia.

NOTE: In our experience, these scooter-board activities have been best demonstrated by a faculty member with the students observing. The activity is then followed by class discussion. We have found the activities to be valuable in relating the laws of motion to gait. Care should be exercised in doing these activities.

a. Stand beside the scooter board and take a vigorous step forward. Next, stand on the scooter board and take a vigorous step forward off the scooter board (expect the scooter board to move backward quickly). Compare your position at the end of each step. Compare the movement of your body and the movement of the scooter board. The movement of the scooter board (the second step), which has a much lower mass than the earth or your body, is significantly greater than the movement of your body (the first step). This is a demonstration of Newton's Second Law of Motion. Explain this in your own words.

b. Place as many weights on the scooter board as you can and still have a place to stand. Now take a vigorous step off the board and note the distance it travels as opposed to the distance of your step. How do these distances compare to the distances seen in a? Write out the equation for Newton's Second Law of Motion in terms of these two activities.

c. Take the weights off the scooter board. Stand on the scooter board and take a *normal* step off as you begin to walk away. Note the distance the scooter board moved. This distance is a reflection of the force needed to get you going from standing still. What law does this activity relate to?

d. Now, place the scooter board in a walkway and walk so that one of your feet steps squarely onto the scooter board during your walking. As you leave the board, note the distance it moves backward during normal gait. This distance reflects the force needed to maintain normal gait. In which case did the board move further back, c or d? Explain why the two distances are different.

*45. Since normal gait is a continuous series of anticipated responses, the ambulator is consistently counting on the reaction force of the ground to propel him. To demonstrate the effect of the ground reaction force working in concert with the coefficient of friction between the foot and the ground, walk straight ahead until you step squarely on the scooter board (as in item 44d above). Immediately make a 90° turn off the foot that is on the scooter board, for example, if you are on your right then turn to the left by pushing off the right. Be prepared for the scooter board to move suddenly and vigorously. The movement of the scooter board is an indicator for the ground reaction force and friction force needed to change directions.

Ground reaction force is an example of which of Newton's laws? Are there any other of the above activities that relate to this same law?

46. During gait, momentum provides considerable force to sustain forward progression. To which of Newton's laws is momentum most directly related?

ANSWERS TO GAIT

1. The two phases of gait are swing and stance phase.

2. | **Traditional** | **RLA** |
   |---|---|
   | Heel strike | Initial contact |
   | Foot flat | Part of loading response |
   | Midstance | Part of midstance |
   | Heel-off | Part of terminal stance |
   | Toe-off | Preswing |
   | Acceleration | Part of initial swing and midswing |
   | Midswing | Part of midswing and terminal swing |
   | Deceleration | Part of terminal swing |

3.

   Figure 11-2

4. a. Heel strike: hip in flexion; knee in full extension; ankle neutral
   b. Foot flat: hip in flexion; knee in slight flexion; ankle in slight plantarflexion
   c. Midstance: hip in slight flexion; knee in extension; ankle in plantarflexion
   d. Heel-off: hip in extension; knee in extension; ankle in dorsiflexion
   e. Toe-off: hip in extension; knee in flexion; ankle in plantarflexion
   f. Acceleration: hip in flexion; knee in flexion; ankle in plantarflexion
   g. Midswing: hip in flexion; knee in flexion; ankle in neutral
   h. Deceleration: hip in flexion; knee in flexion; ankle in neutral

5. The upper-limb movement is in concert with the contralateral lower limb, for example, as the left lower limb moves forward so does the right upper limb. This reciprocal relationship occurs with counter rotation between the shoulder and pelvic girdles.

6. Double support occurs at heel strike and again at toe-off. These periods of double-limb support are the periods of greatest static stability, and as the speed of walking slows, the length of time in double support increases. Patients with decreased balance or stability will naturally tend to walk more slowly.

7. The knee reaches its maximum degree of flexion between toe-off and midswing.

8. Stride length is determined by measuring the distance from the point of heel strike of one extremity to the next heel strike of the same extremity.

9. Stride length is measured in relation to the ipsilateral extremity while step length is measured from heel strike of one extremity to heel strike of the other extremity.

10. The velocity of gait is determined by the number of steps completed per minute multiplied by the step length. This gives the distance covered per minute.

11. As cadence increases, the duration of double support decreases.

*12. The base of support is that area between and under both feet, if both feet are on the floor; or under one foot if it is on the floor alone as in midstance. Therefore, when both feet are on the ground, the drawing of the base of support will include the area between the feet as well as under the feet.

13. The width of the base of support in the child is wider than the adult due to a higher center of gravity (COG) and decreased equilibrium reactions in the child. An elderly adult also has a wider base of support than the younger adult due to the elderly adult's slower gait pattern and slowed reaction time which requires greater static stabilization.

14. There are 7° of normal toe-out during ambulation.
    a. As speed increases, the degree of toe-out decreases.
    b. The greater the degree of toe-out the larger the area of the base of support.
    c. The larger the base of support, the greater the static stability.
    d. There is an inverse relationship between static stability and mobility. As one goes up, the other must go down.
    e. Increased speed requires increased mobility. Increased speed also provides dynamic stability, as in riding a bicycle. As the speed of ambulation goes up, the requirement and usefulness of toe-out goes down.

*15. a. The line between successive heel impressions of the same foot is the reference line against which the angle of toe-out is measured. This is the line of progression. A midline is chosen on the powder footprint, and the goniometer is placed along it and the line of progression. This activity reinforces use of the goniometer as well as solving the problem of where the reference line is drawn in relation to the footprint.
    b. Horizontal lines will have to be drawn across the back of the heel prints in order to measure from one to the other. The horizontals will have to be parallel in order to measure from one foot to the other to obtain step length. This exercise leads to discussion of what effect certain gait abnormalities have on stride versus step length and why.
    Step width is the distance between parallel lines of progression, one for the right and one for the left.

*16. You should feel rotation in the horizontal plane, lateral tilting in the frontal plane, and a lateral shift from one foot to the other.

*17. As the feet become wider apart, the lateral shift will increase in order to get the center of gravity over the stance foot. This increases the lateral excursion of the center of gravity and the energy output.

*18. The rotating pelvis will bring the swinging hip forward placing the foot further in front.

19. The apparent lengthening of the lower limbs by the pelvic rotation serves to diminish the amount of drop of the center of mass for a given step length. Over the same step length but without pelvic rotation, the hips would have to flex and extend further producing a greater vertical excursion in the center of mass.

20. Vertical displacement of the center of gravity creates work and energy expenditure. Lateral movement of the center of gravity creates linear momentum which must be counteracted by muscular effort and thus creates an expenditure of energy.

21. Lack of knee flexion causes compensatory movements such as hip hiking on the affected side or circumducting the affected lower limb to clear the foot off the ground during swing phase. These compensations cause an increase in the vertical displacement of the center of gravity. Lack of knee flexion also disrupts the interaction between the ankle and the knee and the smooth transition to stance. All of this increases the energy cost of gait.

22. The extended stance limb at midstance tends to elevate the center of gravity. The pelvic drop allows the

center of gravity to fall and compensates for the extended midstance limb which has raised the COG. The pelvic drop helps limit the excursion of the center of mass.

23. The angle of inclination, with the femoral head seated in the acetabulum, guides the shaft of the femur toward the midline, thus narrowing the base of support.

24. Physiological valgus at the knee.

25. The transition from swing to stance phase accompanies the transition from a descending to an ascending center of gravity. To smooth that transition, the knee flexes following heel strike and the foot plantar flexes from heel strike to foot flat. This effectively shortens the limb as the center of gravity starts to rise, slowing the rise. The extension of the knee with plantar flexion of the ankle from midstance through heel-off effectively does the reverse, that is, apparently lengthening the stance limb to decrease the descent of the center of gravity since it is now moving downward from its highest elevation at midstance.

26. The determinants of gait include: (1) pelvic rotation in the horizontal plane, (2) lateral pelvic tilt (drop to the unsupported side), (3) knee flexion, (4 & 5) knee with ankle interactions (shortening or lengthening a limb), and (6) physiologic valgus at the knee.

27. The determinants of gait help to minimize vertical rise of the COG, prevent an excessive drop in the body's COG, minimize the side-to-side movement of the COG, and provide a smooth transition to the weight-bearing limb which smooths the movement of the COG in space. All these effects serve to minimize energy expenditure during normal gait.

28. The dorsiflexors of the ankle are most active during heel strike.
    a. Eccentric
    b. Prevents the foot from slapping the ground in the transition from heel strike to foot flat.

29. a. Either dosiflexion or maintenance of neutral.
    b. To slow the dorsiflexion or stabilize the ankle as the line of gravity passes in front of the ankle producing a dorsiflexion moment.
    c. Either eccentric if dorsiflexion is occurring, or isometric if no movement is occurring.

30. At heel strike, the line of gravity and the line of force up the limb from the foot striking the ground fall behind the knee-joint axis producing a flexion moment at the knee. The quadriceps contracts to prevent the knee from buckling.

31. The hamstrings function to decelerate the forward swing of the limb and to prevent excessive hip flexion as well as knee extension due to momentum. They also serve with the gluteus maximus to stabilize the hip at heel strike when the body weight is carried on a flexed hip.

32. The gluteus maximus provides hip control on the stance limb. It may also aid in the forward swing of the contralateral limb.

33. The hip flexors are most active during acceleration and are responsible for the initiation of the swing phase of gait.

34. The abductor muscles function as lateral stabilizers of the pelvis, preventing excessive lowering of the pelvis on the unsupported side during the stance phase of gait. As the pelvis drops, the contraction is eccentric. While the pelvis is stable, the contraction is isometric.

35. The erector spinae muscles are most active during heel strike. The right erector spinae contract when the right heel strikes the ground, and contract again but more strongly when the left heel hits the ground. Since the left erector spinae are performing the reverse of the right, then both contract at each heel strike, but asymmetrically depending upon which heel is hitting the ground. This is due to the muscles acting as trunk stabilizers.

*36. d. The muscles of gait almost continuously contract when you walk slowly because there is no dynamic balance or momentum to keep you up or to keep you moving.

e. Normal gait is propelled to a great extent by momentum (inertia). This force keeps you going if you try to stop quickly.
f. Once the body is moving, short bursts of muscle contraction keep it going. The tendency to fall forward if you stop quickly is a barometer of the force of momentum in gait.

37. The joint motions relying on momentum are the completion of flexion of the humerus at the shoulder, completion of flexion of the femur at the hip in swing phase, extension of the tibia at the knee in swing phase, extension of the femur at the hip in stance phase, completion of extension of the tibia at the knee in stance phase, dorsiflexion of the tibia at the ankle in stance phase. There are at least two sources of momentum, the swinging limbs, primarily the lower limb, and the push-off of the gastrocnemius soleus from heel-off to toe-off.

*38. a. Concentrate on placement of the markers around major joints and on parts having wide excursions of movement. Trial and error a few times will aid in deciding the best locations that assist observation. The one exception is to place a marker on the crest of the tibia and one on the sacrum so rotation of the tibia and pelvis in the horizontal plane can be observed. Hint: The tibial and sacral markers should be a lightweight protrusion such as a drinking straw that is taped onto the part at a right angle so it projects away from the body.
    To evaluate vertical displacement of the center of mass, use a marker on the trunk lateral to the location of the center of mass.
c. Actions of the joints can be confirmed by your kinesiology text.
d. The COG is at its highest at midstance and lowest at double-limb support.

39. Right stride length will be shortened because stance on the left will be prematurely terminated. In order to extend stance on the left, the gastrocnemius-soleus must stabilize the ankle when the line of gravity falls anterior to the joint. This occurs after midstance when the swing leg is moving toward deceleration.

40. Weakness of the tibialis anterior also causes a "steppage gait" during swing phase. In order to clear the toes from the ground, the individual will lift the knee higher than normal using increased hip flexion and possibly increased knee flexion.

41. Other muscles available to assist the tibialis anterior are the other anterior compartment muscles, the extensor digitorum longus, and the extensor hallucis longus.

42. The midtarsal and tarsometatarsal joints can mask a fused talocrural joint.

*43. a. Posterior trunk lurch bilaterally to keep the line of gravity well posterior to the hip
b. Lateral trunk lurch over the stance hip
c. Forward thrust of the pelvis at each toe-off
d. Genu recurvatum at heel strike or press the knee into locked extension with the ipsilateral hand
e. Steppage during swing and foot slap at heel strike
   Demonstration or confirmation by a faculty member is helpful in this activity.

*44. These four activities are self-explained within the context of the item. Review of the three laws of motion assists the discussion, and aids further discussion of how each activity can reflect aspects of each of the laws other than the highlighted one. The activities aid the discussion of the contribution of momentum to the force of locomotion and discussion of the relative force of propulsion of the hip extensors and plantarflexors when overcoming static inertia.

*45. This activity dramatically demonstrates the contribution of the resistance of the ground to the direction and continuation of locomotion. An appreciation should develop that in moving forward or when turning, the body's effort is in a posterior or lateral direction and that it is actually the returned force of the ground that propels the body in the opposite direction.
    This is an example of the third law, the Law of Reaction. While items 44a, b, and c most directly apply to the Law of Acceleration (the second law), they can also be seen as applications of the third law.

46. The Law of Inertia.